POSTPARTUM DEPRESSION

Understanding and Healing from Postpartum Depression for a First-Time Mom

Lorraine Rose

CONTENTS

Hardcover: 979-8-9925167-0-8
Paperback: 979-8-9925167-1-5
Audiobook: 979-8-9925167-2-2
Ebook: 979-8-9925167-3-9
Library of Congress Number: 2-465-561
First edition January 2025
Edited by Lorraine Rose
Cover art by Lorraine Rose
Layout by Lorraine Rose
LTaylor Publishing
https:Ltaylorselfpublishing.com

INTRODUCTION

When my first son was born, I remember sitting on the nursery floor, surrounded by a sea of tiny socks and stuffed animals, feeling completely overwhelmed. I was supposed to feel joy. Instead, there I was, sobbing into a burp cloth, wondering if I was the only mother in the world who didn't have it all together. I felt like I was drowning in a sea of expectations and emotions that no one had warned me about. Postpartum depression crept in quietly, like an unwelcome guest, and before I knew it, it had taken over my life.

This book is my way of reaching out to you, the new mom who might feel lost in the maze of early motherhood. It's here to provide understanding, support, and practical guidance for dealing with postpartum depression. You need to know that it's okay not to be okay. Addressing this often-overlooked aspect of motherhood is crucial. You deserve to feel supported and understood.

I've walked this path as a full-time working mom of two energetic boys. The early days of motherhood were a mix of sleepless nights and constant self-doubt. I tried to juggle work, family, and the overpowering emotions that came with postpartum depression. It wasn't pretty. It wasn't perfect. But it was real. And slowly, I found a way through it by seeking help and allowing myself to accept support.

I want you to know that you are not alone. There are so many new mothers out there feeling isolated, guilty, and overwhelmed. We all share these feelings at some point, and it's okay to admit it. The connection we have is powerful. Knowing that someone else has been there can make all the difference.

Did you know that 1 in 7 women experience postpartum depression? That's a staggering number, yet we often feel like it's something to be ashamed of. We need to change that conversation. We need to bring postpartum depression into the light. It's more common than we think, and there's no shame in seeking help.

This book teaches you to understand your emotions, give yourself grace, and recognize when to seek help. It combines practical advice with emotional support. This isn't just a guide; it's a companion on your journey.

I want to leave you with a message of hope and empowerment. Recovery and self-discovery are not just dreams; they are possible and within reach. You can navigate this challenging time and become stronger on the other side. This book is here to walk with you every step of the way.

So, I invite you to dive into these pages. Engage with the content, use the provided strategies, and join a community of mothers supporting each other through similar experiences. Take this first step toward healing and empowerment. You are not alone, and you are stronger than you know. Let's walk this path together.

CHAPTER 1: UNDERSTANDING POSTPARTUM DEPRESSION

One day, amid the chaos of diaper changes and late-night feedings, I found myself staring at my reflection, wondering who that exhausted, disheveled woman was. She looked vaguely familiar, like a poorly drawn version of the person I used to be. I laughed, not because it was funny, but because sometimes you must laugh to avoid crying. If you've had a similar moment, you're not alone. This chapter is about peeling back the layers of postpartum depression, a topic that often hides in the shadows of new parenthood. Let's face it: the term "baby blues" sounds almost charming, like a cute pair of socks you might buy for your newborn. But what if the blues don't go away? What if they settle in and make themselves at home? There's a world of difference between a fleeting case of the baby blues and the relentless grip of postpartum depression, and understanding that difference is vital.

1.1 Beyond the Baby Blues: Recognizing Postpartum Depression

The baby blues, as whimsical as they sound, are a natural phenomenon that affects up to 80% of new parents. They often sneak up on you a few days after giving birth and can linger for a couple of weeks. You might find yourself crying over spilled milk

—literally—and feeling more irritable than usual. But like a brief rain shower, they tend to pass without leaving much of a mark. In contrast, postpartum depression is more like a storm that refuses to move on. It's not just a temporary dip in your mood; it's a deep trench that can last for months, casting a shadow over what should be joyful moments. The baby blues might make you feel a bit off-kilter, but postpartum depression can hijack your ability to function day-to-day.

Recognizing the signs of postpartum depression is crucial for your well-being. Symptoms such as persistent sadness or a sense of hopelessness can creep in quietly, making everyday tasks feel insurmountable. You might struggle to bond with your baby, even though you love them deeply, which can compound your guilt. Severe anxiety or panic attacks may become unwelcome guests in your already crowded mind. These symptoms are more than just the typical exhaustion of new parenthood; they are red flags that need attention. Understanding these signs can help you take the first steps toward reclaiming your peace of mind.

Identifying postpartum depression early on can lead to better outcomes, much like catching a leaky roof before it ruins the whole house. Early recognition increases the likelihood of successful intervention and can prevent symptoms from worsening over time. It's about grabbing that lifeline before you're too far adrift. The sooner you acknowledge what's happening, the sooner you can start finding your way back to yourself. Seeking help isn't a sign of weakness; it's a brave step toward healing. It's important to remember that you're not charting this course alone. Many mothers have navigated these waters and emerged stronger on the other side.

Postpartum depression is more common than we often acknowledge. As stated previously, nearly 1 in 7 mothers in the U.S. experience it, which means it's happening all around us, even if we don't always talk about it. It's a shared experience that binds us together in understanding. There's a comforting solidarity in knowing that you're not the only one facing these challenges. Knowing that other mothers have stood where you stand now can be a beacon of hope. They've felt the weight of these emotions and, with time and support, have found their way to brighter days. So, let's shed light on postpartum depression, break the silence, and remind ourselves that it's okay to ask for help when we need it. You're not alone in this, and together, we can navigate the path to healing with empathy and strength.

1.2 The Emotional Rollercoaster: Understanding Your Feelings

Picture this: you're holding your newborn, a bundle of possibilities and dreams, and your heart swells with a joy so pure it feels like it might burst. Then, in the blink of an eye, that joy is shadowed by a creeping anxiety. What if you're not enough? What if you miss a sign, a cry for help, a need unmet? These swings between excitement and fear can feel like you're on a carnival ride with no off switch. Add in the overwhelming love and the fierce instinct to protect this little being, and you've got a cocktail of emotions that can leave you breathless. It's an emotional rollercoaster, and you're not the only one on it. Every new mother has felt the dizzying highs and lows, the moments of pure bliss mingled with the shadows of doubt. It's all part of the chaotic symphony of new motherhood.

The fact is, your emotions aren't just acting up for no reason. They're responding to a massive hormonal shift happening in your body. Imagine your hormones as the conductors of your emotional orchestra. During pregnancy, they're all about nurturing and preparing. But after childbirth, there's a sudden drop in estrogen and progesterone, the hormones that have been keeping things in symphony. This abrupt change can throw your neurotransmitters, those tiny messengers in your brain, into disarray. It's like they've been handed a new script with no rehearsal time. The result? Mood swings, anxiety, and that persistent feeling of being off-balance. It's a lot to handle, especially when you're trying to keep it together for your new family.

And then there's the sleep deprivation, the unsung villain of postpartum life. You start to feel like a zombie, shuffling through the days in a haze. Interrupted sleep cycles aren't just tiring; they're destabilizing. They rob you of the mental clarity you need to navigate the emotional landscape of motherhood. This lack of sleep can amplify mood swings, making minor issues feel like insurmountable obstacles. You might cry over the most minor things, like when I burst into tears because I couldn't find the matching sock for my baby's outfit. Sleep deprivation is more than just an inconvenience; it's a thief that steals your peace of mind.

It's important to remember that these emotions, as overwhelming and contradictory as they may seem, are valid. They're a testament to the incredible changes you're going through. Accepting that it's okay to feel a mix of joy, fear, and love can be liberating. You're not failing; you're feeling. Many mothers have shared how they felt swept away by their emotions, only to find solace in knowing they weren't alone. A mental health professional once told me, "Your feelings are like waves—they ebb and flow, but they don't define you." It's a reminder that emotions are transient, even the ones that feel like they've set up camp in your heart.

So, as you navigate this emotional rollercoaster, remember that it's okay to ride the waves. It's okay to have moments where you feel like you're on top of the world and others where you're not so sure. This is your story, and every emotion is a part of it. You're stronger than you know, and every day is a step forward.

1.3 The Science Behind PPD: Hormonal and Biological Factors

After giving birth, it feels like your body has just run a marathon, climbed Everest, and completed an Ironman all at once. But the real upheaval is happening inside, where your hormones are having a party—only you weren't invited. During pregnancy, your body is flooded with hormones like estrogen and progesterone, which help create the perfect environment for your baby. It's like a hormonal symphony, playing a lullaby that keeps everything in balance. But after childbirth, this symphony comes to a screeching halt. The levels of these hormones plummet, leaving your body scrambling to adjust to a new normal. Imagine it like a rollercoaster ride where the climb is long and steady, but the drop is sudden and steep. This dramatic decline can leave you feeling all sorts of out of sync.

The thyroid, a small but mighty gland in your neck, can also throw its hat into the ring. It regulates energy levels and metabolism and can go haywire after childbirth. Some women may experience a thyroid hormone imbalance that mimics or exacerbates symptoms of depression. You might feel sluggish or anxious without knowing why. It's like your body has a mind of its own, and you're left trying to catch up. Understanding these biological changes can help you realize that what you're feeling has a basis in science, not just emotions.

Meanwhile, your brain is dealing with its own set of challenges. Neurochemical changes are the behind-the-scenes players that can contribute to postpartum depression. Serotonin and dopamine, neurotransmitters often called the "feel-good" chemicals, can be out of whack. When these chemicals are imbalanced, it can lead to sadness or lack of motivation. Think of it as a dimmer switch turned down on your brain's ability to feel joy or satisfaction. It's not that you don't want to feel those things; it's that your brain isn't making it easy.

Genetics also plays a part in this complex picture. Some women are more predisposed to postpartum depression due to genetic factors. Research has shown that certain genetic markers can increase susceptibility. It's a bit like a lottery; sometimes, the cards are stacked against you. However, knowing that genetics can play a role helps remove the stigma. It's not a reflection of your strength or character but rather a part of your biological makeup. Recognizing this can be a step forward in understanding and managing postpartum depression.

Many refer to the postpartum period as the "fourth trimester," a continuation of pregnancy that is often overlooked. This is a time when both mother and baby are still adjusting to life outside the womb. The demands are high, and the support often needs to be improved. Society tends to celebrate the birth and then swiftly move on, leaving mothers to navigate this critical time with less guidance. The fourth trimester is about healing, bonding, and adjusting, yet societal expectations can make these tasks feel insurmountable. You're expected to bounce back, both physically and emotionally, as if nothing monumental just happened.

Understanding the science behind postpartum depression can be both enlightening and reassuring. It's not just "all in your head" or something you can shake off with sheer willpower. It's a natural, biological response to an incredible life change. Knowing what's happening inside your body can empower you to seek the care and support you need. You're not alone; there's no shame in needing help navigating this complex time.

1.4 Dispelling Myths: What Postpartum Depression is Not

Let's start by tackling a myth that's as persistent as a toddler demanding candy before dinner: the idea that experiencing postpartum depression (PPD) is a sign of weakness. It's a notion that society loves to cling to, as if admitting to these struggles somehow diminishes your worth as a mother. But let's be honest —PPD is not a reflection of your strength or character. It's a medical condition, not a personal failing. Society has long pushed an unrealistic narrative that mothers should seamlessly transition into their new roles with a smile plastered on their faces, no matter the chaos swirling around them. This stigma can make reaching out for help feel like shouting into a void. It's crucial to recognize this pressure for what it is: unfounded and harmful. You wouldn't blame yourself for catching the flu, so why should mental health be any different? Embracing this understanding is the first step toward breaking free from the shackles of shame and seeking the support you deserve.

Now, let's bust another myth wide open: the belief that postpartum depression only affects a select few. This misconception couldn't be further from the truth. PPD doesn't discriminate. It doesn't care about your age, race, or socioeconomic status. It can touch the lives of any new mother. You might be a young mom fresh out of college or a seasoned professional who thought she had everything under control. PPD can still find its way in. I've heard stories from mothers of all backgrounds, from those living in bustling cities to those in quiet rural areas. The common thread is the feeling of being blindsided by something they didn't think could happen to them. Recognizing that PPD can affect any mother helps dismantle the myth that it's confined to a specific group. It's more prevalent than society lets on, and acknowledging this can foster empathy and understanding among us all.

There's also the misguided notion that postpartum depression means you don't love your baby. This is perhaps the most heartbreaking myth, as it can exacerbate feelings of guilt and inadequacy. The truth is that bonding issues are just one aspect of PPD, and they don't define the depth of your love for your child. Bonding and attachment are complex processes that can be influenced by many factors, including your mental health. It's possible to love your baby fiercely while still struggling to connect emotionally as you imagined you would. It's important to differentiate between these bonding challenges and attachment disorders, which are separate issues requiring different approaches. Your love isn't diminished by the struggles you face.

Instead, it's a testament to your resilience and commitment to your baby's well-being.

Finally, let's put to rest the dangerous idea that postpartum depression will resolve on its own. This misconception can lead to unnecessary suffering and prevent mothers from seeking the help they truly need. Untreated PPD can have serious consequences, not just for you but also for your family. It can affect your ability to care for yourself and your baby, potentially impacting your long-term mental health. Treatment is crucial, whether through therapy, medication, or support groups. Much like tending to a garden, addressing PPD requires nurturing and care to foster growth and healing. Ignoring it won't make it disappear. It's about taking proactive steps to safeguard your mental health and embrace the support available to you. Seeking treatment isn't a sign of defeat; it's an act of courage and love for yourself and your family.

1.5 Common Misconceptions: Separating Fact from Fiction

Let's unravel these common misconceptions that seem to cling to postpartum depression, like gum on a shoe. First up is the idea that postpartum depression is the same as postpartum psychosis. The two conditions are as different as night and day. Postpartum depression is a serious but manageable condition characterized by persistent sadness, anxiety, and fatigue. It affects many mothers, but it doesn't usually include the severe symptoms seen in postpartum psychosis. Postpartum psychosis, on the other hand, is a rare and severe mental illness. It can consist of hallucinations, delusions, and paranoia. While both require attention, their severity and treatment differ significantly. Postpartum depression often responds well to therapy and medication, leading to recovery for many. Postpartum psychosis, however, requires immediate medical intervention, often including hospitalization. Understanding these differences helps us approach each condition with the appropriate care and concern.

There's also a persistent and damaging myth that all mothers with postpartum depression are at risk of harming their children. This couldn't be further from the truth. While intrusive thoughts can occur, they don't define the experience for most women with postpartum depression. According to the data, the likelihood of harm is relatively low. It's crucial to balance this understanding with recognizing that professional assessment is essential. Mental health professionals can provide the proper support and guidance, ensuring safety and well-being for both mother and child.

Another myth that needs busting is the idea that treatment options for postpartum depression are limited or ineffective. The truth is there's a wide range of treatments available that can be tailored to individual needs. Therapy and counseling can be incredibly beneficial, offering a safe space to explore emotions and develop coping strategies. Cognitive-behavioral therapy (CBT) is particularly effective in helping mothers reframe negative thought patterns. Medication, such as antidepressants, can also play a crucial role in treatment, especially when therapy alone isn't enough. The key is finding the right balance and approach that works for each individual. It's about opening the door to possibilities and finding the support that leads to healing.

Finally, let's tackle the misconception that postpartum depression only occurs immediately after birth. In reality, postpartum depression can develop anytime within the first year after childbirth. It's not just a phenomenon of the early weeks; it can sneak up on you when you least expect it. Factors such as lack of support, ongoing stress, and hormonal changes can contribute to a delayed onset. It's like a slow-burning candle that suddenly flares up when the conditions are right. Recognizing that postpartum depression can appear later on is important for both mothers and their support systems. It encourages ongoing vigilance and support throughout the first year, ensuring that help is available whenever it's needed.

In closing, let's remind ourselves that understanding these misconceptions is a powerful step toward change. By separating fact from fiction, we can pursue a path forward with clarity and compassion. Whether you're reaching out for help, supporting a loved one, or simply seeking to understand, knowledge is your ally. You're not walking this path alone. Together, we can foster an environment where every mother feels seen, heard, and supported—free from stigma and full of hope.

CHAPTER 2: IDENTIFYING SYMPTOMS AND SEEKING HELP

You know that feeling when you're trying to find a lost sock and somehow end up cleaning the entire closet? That's what self-assessment feels like. You start with a tiny step, and suddenly, you're unraveling layers you didn't even know you had. But here's the thing: when it comes to postpartum depression, self-awareness is your best buddy. It's like tuning into your own personal radar system. You can catch those little blips on the screen before they grow into full-blown storms. The key is honest reflection. This isn't about beating yourself up for feeling off; it's about recognizing that something isn't quite right and deciding to do something about it. Early detection is like catching a leaky faucet before it becomes a flooded basement. You can save yourself a lot of heartache down the line.

How do you know if what you're experiencing is more than just a rough patch? Here's a checklist to help you figure it out. Emotional symptoms are the usual suspects: persistent sadness that lingers like an uninvited guest, overwhelming anxiety that makes even simple tasks feel monumental, and irritability that snaps at those closest to you. On the physical side, there's fatigue that no amount of coffee can fix and sleep disturbances that make you feel like you're in a never-ending cycle of exhaustion. Behaviorally, you might withdraw from social interactions, even with people you love, as if you've forgotten how to connect. If you're ticking more than a few boxes, it might be time to look closely at these feelings.

Consider keeping a mood-tracking journal. Think of it as a diary for your emotions. Each day, jot down how you're feeling, what you're thinking, and any physical symptoms you notice. Over time, patterns emerge. Maybe Mondays are particularly tough, or specific interactions leave you feeling drained. These insights are like breadcrumbs leading you back to yourself. Daily mood-tracking templates can be as simple as jotting down a few words or as detailed as you like. As you document your days, you might notice that what seems like an off day is actually part of a recurring pattern. Identifying these patterns can be incredibly revealing and empowering.

2.1 Mood Tracking Exercise

Start each day by writing down your baseline mood. Are you waking up feeling refreshed, anxious, or somewhere in between? Note any significant events or interactions that might have influenced your mood. At the end of the day, reflect on how you feel compared to the morning. This exercise can help illuminate patterns and triggers, providing valuable insights into your emotional landscape.

Another tool to consider is comparing your current feelings with your pre-pregnancy emotional state. Remember when you used to feel like you had it all together? Or at least most of it? Use that as your baseline. It's not about longing for the past but understanding how your emotional landscape has shifted. Maybe you used to bounce back quickly after a bad day, but now those days stretch into weeks. Changes in coping mechanisms are worth noting, too. If your usual stress relievers aren't cutting it anymore, that's a sign that something deeper might be at play.

So, as you navigate these early days of motherhood, remember that self-assessment is not about judgment. It's about curiosity and compassion. It's about giving yourself the grace to say, "Okay, this is where I'm at. What do I need to do to take care of myself?" You're not alone in this, and recognizing the signs in yourself is a decisive first step toward finding the support and relief you deserve. Trust that you have the strength and wisdom to face whatever comes your way.

2.2 When to Seek Help: Navigating the Decision-Making Process

Imagine this: you've felt like you're wading through molasses, your emotions heavy and unyielding, for weeks. When do you decide that it's time to seek help? This decision can feel daunting, but understanding when professional help is necessary can make it more straightforward. Start by considering the duration and severity of your symptoms. If those feelings of sadness or anxiety have been your constant companions for more than two weeks, it's a sign that you might need extra support.

Similarly, if these emotions are so intense that they impact your daily functioning—making it difficult to care for your baby or maintain relationships—it's time to reach out. It's not just about the presence of symptoms but how they affect your life. If you cannot get out of bed or your relationships with loved ones are now strained, these are red flags. Your well-being is important, and addressing these issues early can prevent them from snowballing into something more overwhelming.

But let's be honest; seeking help is more complex than it sounds. There are barriers, big and small, that can make it feel like climbing a mountain. One of the biggest hurdles is the stigma surrounding mental health. You might worry that seeking help means you've failed as a mother or that others will judge you. These fears are powerful, but they shouldn't hold you back. Logistical challenges, like finding childcare or fitting appointments into an already packed schedule, can also be daunting. It's like trying to play Tetris with your time, and sometimes it feels like there's not enough space. Recognizing these challenges is essential, but letting them stop you is not. It's about finding ways to navigate them, like enlisting the help of a friend or family member to watch the baby for a few hours. Your health is worth the effort, even if it means asking for help in unexpected ways.

Once you've decided to seek help, the next step is taking action. This might seem like a mountain of its own, but breaking it down into smaller steps can make it manageable. Start by making a list of healthcare providers. Look for therapists or doctors who specialize in postpartum depression or women's mental health. Your OB-GYN might have recommendations, or you can explore online directories. Once you have a list, prepare some questions to ask them. Consider what you need from a provider: Do you prefer a therapist offering online sessions? Are you looking for someone with specific experience in postpartum issues? Preparing these questions can help you feel more in control and ensure you find the right fit for your needs.

Early intervention is a gift to yourself. Seeking help sooner rather than later can lead to improved recovery rates, giving you a better chance at regaining your footing. It can also enhance your family dynamics, as you can better engage and connect with your loved ones. Imagine being able to enjoy moments with your baby, free from the weight of depression. This is possible when you take those initial steps toward getting the support you need. The benefits of early intervention are real and significant. It's about giving yourself the best chance to thrive, not just survive. So, while the process may feel overwhelming, remember that each step you take is a step toward healing. You're doing this for yourself and for your family.

2.3 Overcoming Fear of Judgment: Opening Up About Your Experience

Let's face it: the fear of being judged can feel like the elephant in the room, and for new moms grappling with postpartum depression, it often feels like the elephant is doing a tap dance on your chest. The worry that you might be perceived as a "bad mother" looms large. It's a fear fed by societal expectations and that nagging little voice in your head that says you should be able to handle this. But here's the truth: you're not a bad mom for needing help. You're human. And humans, even the best of them, need support sometimes. Anxiety about how others perceive you —whether it's your family, friends, or the community—can hold you back from sharing your struggles. These fears are authentic and valid, but they shouldn't silence you. Remember, everyone's got their stuff, and yours just happens to come with a side of diapers and sleepless nights.

Opening up about your experience might feel like stepping into a spotlight, but it doesn't have to be all at once. Easing into conversations can make the process more manageable. Start by practicing what you want to say to someone you trust. This could be your partner, a close friend, or even your reflection in the mirror. Practicing can help you untangle your thoughts and find the right words. If words fail you in the moment, consider using scripted dialogues as a guide. Something as simple as, "I've been feeling overwhelmed, and I think it's more than just the baby blues," can open the door to deeper discussions. It's about finding and using your voice, even if it initially feels shaky.

Vulnerability, often seen as a weakness, is actually one of your greatest strengths. When you share your struggles, you lighten your load and permit others to do the same. Think of it as a ripple effect of honesty and connection. There are countless stories of women who found healing in their openness. One mom described how sharing her postpartum depression with a friend led to a deeper bond and mutual support. Another found peace in a support group, realizing she wasn't the only one feeling adrift. The act of sharing is powerful. It transforms isolation into community and fear into understanding. You might be surprised by the compassion and support you receive when you let others in.

Support groups can be a haven for fostering acceptance. In these spaces, you're among others who get it—people who won't flinch at your raw honesty. Whether it's a local group that meets in a cozy community center or an online group you join from the comfort of your couch, these settings offer a safe place to express yourself without fear of judgment. Participants often speak of the relief they felt upon realizing they weren't alone. Testimonials from group members reflect a shared sense of belonging, a feeling of being seen and heard. These groups can be lifelines, offering camaraderie, practical advice, and emotional support. They remind you that you are part of a larger community, one that acknowledges your struggle and celebrates your courage.

So, while the fear of judgment might feel like a looming shadow, remember that openness is a light that can dissipate it. You are not alone in your experiences; sharing them will pave the way for healing—not just for yourself but for anyone fortunate enough to hear your truth.

2.4 Professional vs. Peer Support: Finding What Works for You

Navigating postpartum depression can sometimes feel like you're lost in a forest without a map, and deciding between professional and peer support can be like choosing between two paths. Professional support offers the clinical expertise that can be crucial when dealing with more severe symptoms. Therapists and counselors are trained to help you untangle the complex emotions that come with postpartum depression. They can provide structured therapy sessions, such as cognitive-behavioral therapy, which are designed to provide you with coping mechanisms and a deeper understanding of what's happening in your mind. It's like having a guide who knows the terrain and can offer practical tools to handle those steep climbs.

On the other hand, peer support is like sitting around a cozy campfire with others who've been through the same forest. These are the people who know firsthand what it feels like to be in the thick of postpartum depression. They've waded through the same emotional underbrush and can offer empathy and camaraderie that's hard to find elsewhere. Sharing experiences with peers can be incredibly validating. It's comforting to hear " Me too" and know that someone else truly understands it. Peer support groups, whether in person or online, provide a space where you can voice your fears, share your victories, and be heard without judgment. The shared experience of motherhood creates a bond that can be healing and empowering.

There's also the potential for a hybrid approach that combines the best of both worlds. You don't have to choose one path exclusively. Many find it beneficial to alternate between therapy sessions with a professional and meetings with a peer support group. This way, you benefit from the expert guidance of a therapist while also gaining the warmth and solidarity that only peers can provide. Creating a balanced support schedule that incorporates both types of support can offer a more comprehensive approach to managing postpartum depression. You might feel like you're covering all your bases, ensuring you have the emotional and practical support you need.

Cultural factors can play a big role in choosing the right type of support as well. Your cultural background might influence your preferences regarding mental health care. Some cultures have specific views on mental health that can shape how you feel about seeking professional help versus peer support. It's important to find resources that respect and understand your cultural needs. Look for culturally sensitive therapists trained to incorporate cultural considerations into their practice. This can help bridge the gap between traditional mental health treatments and cultural beliefs, making the process more comfortable and practical.

Finding the right support network can feel daunting, but there are resources to help you along the way. Directories of therapists who specialize in postpartum issues are a good starting point. Websites and organizations dedicated to women's mental health often have lists of qualified professionals. Online forums for new mothers are also valuable. They offer a platform where you can connect with others, share experiences, and gain insight into different forms of support available to you. These forums can be a treasure trove of information and encouragement, reminding you that you're part of a community that truly understands what you're going through.

2.5 The First Steps: Making Your First Appointment

Setting up that first appointment might seem like a Herculean task but breaking it down into smaller steps can make it more manageable. Think of it as planning a mini getaway, except instead of sun and sand, you're looking for peace of mind. Start by finding the right healthcare provider. This might be a therapist, a psychiatrist, or even your family doctor. You're looking for someone with experience in postpartum depression, someone who speaks the language of motherhood. Think of it like choosing a co-pilot for your flight—someone who knows the skies you're navigating. Recommendations from friends or online reviews can be helpful, but ultimately, you want someone you feel comfortable with. Once you've zeroed in on a few options, give them a call. Yes, the phone can feel like a hundred-pound weight, but it's the first step toward feeling lighter.

Next, let's talk about understanding insurance and payment options. It's not the most glamorous part of the process, but it's necessary. Check with your insurance provider to see what mental health services are covered. Some plans offer a list of in-network providers, saving you a hefty bill later. If you're uninsured, don't panic—there are sliding-scale options and community services that can accommodate different financial situations. It's like looking for the best deal on a flight; a little research can save you a lot of stress. Once you're armed with this information, you're ready to take the plunge and schedule that initial appointment.

What should you expect during this first visit? Picture it as a first date, where you're getting to know someone who can help you untangle your thoughts. The professional will ask a series of questions to understand your situation better. These might cover your symptoms, how long you've been experiencing them, and their impact on your daily life. This is not an interrogation; it's more like a guided conversation to paint the complete picture. You might also complete some paperwork detailing your medical history and any previous treatments. Initial assessments help create a treatment plan tailored to your needs. Setting goals for treatment is an integral part of this process. Maybe you want to feel more connected to your baby, or perhaps you're hoping to manage anxiety better. Whatever your goals, they're valid, and your healthcare provider is there to help you achieve them.

Now, onto the not-so-fun but a crucial part: follow-through. Committing to the treatment process means scheduling regular follow-up appointments. Think of it like brushing your teeth—not always exciting, but necessary for maintaining health. Progress tracking is critical. Some days, it might feel like you're going backward, but these small steps add to significant change over time. Regular check-ins with your provider allow you to assess what's working and what might need a tweak. It's about building a relationship where you feel safe and supported, not just checking off boxes on a to-do list.

Let's address a common concern: confidentiality and privacy. Sharing personal information can feel like handing over your diary, but rest assured, healthcare providers are bound by laws to protect your privacy. They're like vaults, safeguarding your secrets with the utmost care. Understanding the legal aspects of patient confidentiality can ease your mind. Building trust with your provider is a two-way street. It's about creating a space where you feel comfortable being honest about your struggles and triumphs. Your story is yours to share, and they're there to listen without judgment.

Taking these first steps toward seeking help can feel like climbing a steep hill, but remember, you're not doing it alone. You're investing in your well-being, in your ability to be present for yourself and your loved ones. As you navigate this path, remember that every step forward is a victory, no matter how small it seems. So, take a deep breath, pick up that phone, and make the call. Your future self will thank you. Every step you take is a testament to your strength and resilience. It's about finding the support you need to thrive, not just survive.

As you embrace this new chapter of taking care of yourself, remember that this is just the beginning of your journey toward healing. Next, we'll explore how to build a supportive network, harnessing the power of community and connection to lift you up. You're not in this alone, and together, we'll uncover the resources and relationships that will support you every step of the way.

CHAPTER 3: BUILDING A SUPPORTIVE NETWORK

I magine for a moment you're at the center of a vibrant, colorful quilt. Each patch represents someone in your life, stitched together to form a tapestry of support and love. Now, imagine trying to keep warm with only a single patch. Not quite as comforting, right? As you navigate the complexities of postpartum depression, this quilt of support becomes essential —not just one square but the whole, cozy ensemble. A diverse support network is like that quilt, offering warmth and security from all angles. Friends, family, healthcare providers—they all have roles to play in wrapping you in care and understanding.

Friends often provide the emotional support that feels like a lifeline. They're the ones who show up with ice cream when you need a shoulder to cry on or send a text at the perfect moment to remind you that you're not alone. Their empathy and understanding can be a balm, helping you weather the emotional ups and downs. Family, on the other hand, can be pillars of practical support. They might lend a hand with childcare or take on household chores when you need a break. There's something about knowing that someone's got your back, whether it's folding laundry or just being present, that can lighten the load. And let's not forget the professionals—the doctors, therapists, and counselors who offer guidance and expertise. They're the navigators on this journey, helping you make sense of the emotional terrain and providing tools to cope.

But how do you identify who fits into this support network? It starts with recognizing those who show up when you need them most. Trustworthy, empathetic individuals are like the sturdy threads in your quilt, ensuring it holds together. Look for friends and family members who have shown reliability in the past, those who listen without judgment and offer help without strings attached. Assess their availability and willingness to help. Remember, it's not about quantity but quality. A few reliable people can be more supportive than a crowd of acquaintances.

Open communication is the glue that holds these connections together. Without clear communication, even the most willing support network can falter. It's important to discuss your needs and expectations openly. Let your loved ones know what kind of support you're seeking. It could be a weekly coffee date with a friend or having a family member babysit for an hour while you take a much-needed nap. Being specific about your needs helps avoid misunderstandings and ensures that the support you receive is genuinely beneficial. It's also crucial to set boundaries and understand limitations. Not everyone can be available 24/7, and that's okay. Knowing each person's capacity can help you manage expectations and avoid feelings of disappointment.

Once you've established these relationships, nurturing them is vital. Regular check-ins and updates keep the lines of communication open and maintain the strength of your support network. A simple text or phone call can reaffirm your connection and remind your friends and family that their support matters. Expressing gratitude and appreciation goes a long way in solidifying these bonds. A heartfelt thank-you note or a small token of appreciation can convey how much their support means to you. It's about creating a reciprocal relationship where both parties feel valued and understood.

3.1 Support Network Reflection

Take a moment to reflect on your current support system. Who are the key players, and how do they contribute to your well-being? Consider reaching out to these individuals with a note of appreciation, acknowledging their support, and expressing gratitude for their presence in your life.

Building and maintaining a supportive network is not just about seeking help; it's about creating a community woven together with care and understanding. With the right mix of emotional, practical, and professional support, you can face the challenges of postpartum depression with resilience and hope.

3.2 The Role of Partners: Engaging Your Partner in Your Journey

Partners have a unique way of being both your biggest cheerleader and your co-pilot during the bumpy flight of postpartum life. They're the ones who can offer that reassuring squeeze of the hand when things feel overwhelming or whisper those magical words, "You're doing great." Emotional reassurance from your partner can be like a beacon in the fog. It reminds you that you're not in this alone and have someone who's got your back, no matter how messy things get. Sharing parenting responsibilities can also be a game changer. It's about dividing and conquering those never-ending tasks: diaper changes, midnight feedings, and the elusive art of getting the baby to sleep. By working together, you're lightening the load and building a more profound sense of partnership that can strengthen your relationship.

Communication is the secret sauce that keeps this partnership dynamic and effective. It's easy to assume that your partner knows what you need, but the truth is, no one's a mind reader. Regularly scheduled check-ins can make a world of difference. Set aside time to talk, really talk, about how you're both feeling and what you might need from each other. Using "I" statements to express feelings can help avoid the blame game. Instead of saying, "You never help with the baby," try, "I feel overwhelmed when I don't get a break." It's a subtle shift but opens up the conversation without putting your partner on the defensive. These conversations can foster a deeper understanding and help you both feel more connected.

Shared activities can be the glue that binds you together during this chaotic time. Consider taking a co-parenting class or attending a workshop. These experiences can provide valuable insights and give you both a chance to bond over shared learning. Plus, it's like returning to school together, but with less math and more baby talk. Setting aside time for couple bonding is equally essential. Whether it's a weekly date night, a stroll around the block, or simply cuddling on the couch once the baby is asleep, these moments of connection can remind you why you're in this together. They help keep the romance alive, even when life is all about spit-up and sleepless nights.

Of course, every partnership faces challenges, and parenting can amplify them. Differing expectations about parenting roles or how to handle certain situations might arise. It's essential to address these differences head-on rather than letting them fester. Discuss what each of you envisions in your parenting roles and find common ground. Couples counseling might be a helpful resource if these conversations hit a wall. Seeking professional guidance doesn't mean your relationship is failing; it's a proactive step to strengthen it. Counselors can offer a neutral space to navigate tricky topics and provide strategies to improve communication and understanding.

Engaging your partner in your postpartum experience isn't just about sharing tasks; it's about building a team. It's about recognizing that both of you are navigating uncharted waters and are stronger together. A supportive partner can be your anchor, helping you weather the storms of new parenthood with love and resilience. Remember, you're not only partners in parenting but in life. Together, you can create a nurturing environment for your relationship and growing family.

3.3 Finding Your Mama Tribe: Connecting with Other Moms

There's something almost magical about connecting with fellow mothers who get it. It's like you've entered a secret club where everyone speaks the same language and comprehends the unspoken rules. They know the joy of a baby's first giggle and the exhaustion of sleepless nights. Being part of a mom group can offer a sense of validation that's hard to find elsewhere. Suddenly, those overwhelming feelings make sense. In these groups, the shared understanding creates a safe space to express emotions without fear of judgment. You find yourself nodding as someone describes a day that sounds eerily similar to yours. It's more than just camaraderie; it's a lifeline of empathy and support. Not only do you find solace in shared experiences, but there's also a treasure trove of advice and parenting tips to be discovered. Whether it's how to soothe a colicky baby or manage the chaos of mealtime, the collective wisdom of these groups is invaluable. Each mom brings her unique insights, and together, you tackle the challenges of motherhood, one shared story at a time.

Finding your mama tribe might feel like searching for a needle in a haystack, but there are plenty of places to start your search. Local community centers and libraries often host mom groups or parenting classes. These gatherings can be a great way to meet other mothers in your area who are looking for the same connection and support. Don't be afraid to show up and introduce yourself; everyone's there for the same reason. Social media also offers a wealth of opportunities to connect with other moms. Platforms like Facebook have groups dedicated to mothers or those with shared interests in specific locations. Online forums provide a space to exchange experiences and support from the comfort of your home. It's like having a virtual circle of friends who are always there, no matter the hour. Apps like Peanut

(SOURCE 3) can also help you discover and connect with like-minded women nearby, making it easier to find your tribe.

Once you've found a group that feels like a good fit, it's time to dive in. Participating in group activities can deepen your connections and create lasting friendships. Attend regular meet-ups, whether weekly coffee dates or monthly playdates at the park. These gatherings are more than just social events; they're opportunities to learn, laugh, and lean on each other. Joining group challenges or projects can also strengthen your bond with fellow moms. Whether it's a book club or a fitness challenge, working toward a common goal fosters a sense of unity and accomplishment. Plus, it's fun to break out of the daily routine and try something new. Engaging with the group actively helps build a network of support that extends beyond the confines of organized meetings.

Diversity is a crucial element of any thriving community, and mom groups are no different. Embracing various perspectives and backgrounds enriches the group's dynamic and offers invaluable learning opportunities. It's fascinating to discover how different cultural parenting practices can influence the way we raise our children. Sharing these diverse approaches can lead to innovative solutions and broaden your understanding of motherhood. Building a broad support network that includes mothers from various walks of life can also prepare you for the unexpected challenges that arise on this adventure. Each mother's story adds a unique thread to the tapestry of your tribe, weaving together a rich and varied fabric of experiences and insights. This diversity enhances the support you receive and encourages personal growth and a deeper appreciation for the myriad ways mothers navigate the world.

3.4 Utilizing Technology: Online Communities and Resources

Envision this: it's 3 AM, you're up for the third time, and your phone is your lifeline to the outside world. In those moments, technology can be a powerful ally. It's not just about scrolling through social media; it's about tapping into a network of support that's just a click away. Apps focused on mental health tracking can be incredibly helpful. They allow you to monitor your mood and symptoms, providing insights that can inform your discussions with healthcare providers. These apps become a digital diary, capturing the subtle shifts in your emotional landscape that might otherwise go unnoticed. Virtual support groups offer a space to connect with others who are walking similar paths, providing comfort and solidarity when you need it most. The beauty of these groups is that they're available whenever you are, offering advice, empathy, or just a listening ear during those long, sleepless nights.

When seeking out online resources, it's crucial to play detective. Not everything you read on the internet is reliable or helpful. Verify the credibility of information before you accept it as truth. Look for resources backed by reputable organizations or experts in the field. Avoid harmful or toxic communities that might offer unsound advice or foster unhealthy comparisons. These spaces should uplift, not drag you down. It's about finding those corners of the internet where you feel supported and seen.

Engaging online requires a balance that can be tricky to strike. Setting boundaries for screen time is one way to ensure that your digital interactions remain positive. It's easy to fall down the rabbit hole of endless scrolling, but too much screen time can be overwhelming. Establish limits that allow you to connect without becoming consumed. Engaging in moderated forums can also help maintain a positive experience. These platforms often have guidelines to ensure respectful and supportive interactions, creating a safe space for sharing and learning.

One of the most empowering aspects of online communities is the anonymity they can provide. It's like wearing a mask at a costume party, allowing you to express yourself without fear of judgment. This anonymity can be liberating, especially when discussing sensitive topics like postpartum depression. It will enable you to share your experiences openly, knowing your identity is protected. You can access a global perspective through these anonymous interactions, learning from mothers in different cultures and contexts. This broadens your understanding and offers fresh insights into your own experiences. Technology bridges the gap between isolation and connection, offering a lifeline to a world of support and understanding.

Online Resource Checklist

Before diving into any online community or resource, consider these quick checks: Is the source reliable and backed by experts? Are the community guidelines focused on creating a supportive environment? Does the platform offer anonymity, if desired? Ensuring these elements can enhance your online experience and provide the support you seek.

3.5 Involving Relatives: How Family Can Help

Imagine a bustling kitchen where the aroma of a home-cooked meal mingles with the laughter of family. That warmth and support can extend into your postpartum recovery, with relatives playing a pivotal role. They can be your allies in navigating the early days of motherhood, lending a hand with childcare, or tackling household chores that seem endless. Picture your parents or siblings taking the baby for a stroll, giving you a moment to rest, or perhaps combating that mountain of laundry that's been giving you the side-eye all week. Their presence can also provide emotional support and companionship when you need it most. A heartfelt chat over a cup of tea can be a balm for the soul, offering perspective and reassurance that you're not alone in this.

Setting clear expectations with family is crucial for a harmonious support system. It's like drawing up a playbook for everyone involved, ensuring everyone knows their role and responsibilities. Start by outlining specific tasks that would be most helpful. Maybe it's your sister bringing over groceries once a week or your dad fixing that creaky door that's been driving you up the wall. Be clear about what you need so there's no room for misunderstanding. Discussing privacy and personal boundaries is equally important. Let your family know when you need space or time alone, and reassure them that it's nothing personal. It's all about building an atmosphere where everyone feels comfortable and respected. These conversations might initially feel awkward, but they're essential for maintaining healthy relationships and avoiding unnecessary friction.

Family involvement can come with its own set of challenges. Differing parenting opinions might rear their heads with well-meaning advice that doesn't quite align with your approach. Aunt Kathy's insistence on letting the baby "cry it out" might not sit well with your soothing techniques. Balancing these opinions with your instincts can be tricky. Standing firm in your parenting choices is important while remaining open to suggestions that resonate with you. Finding a balance between family visits and personal space can also be a juggling act. While you appreciate their company, you also need time to bond as a nuclear family. It's okay to set limits on visits and to carve out time for just you and your baby. Remember, it's your family, your rules.

Involving family in a structured support plan can enhance their contribution to your recovery. Consider organizing family meetings to discuss support roles, ensuring everyone is on the same page. Approach these meetings as collaborative decision-making sessions where each person's input is valued. Perhaps one family member takes on the role of organizing meals while another coordinates childcare during the week. This structured approach can prevent overlap and ensure that support is evenly distributed. It's like running a well-oiled machine, where everyone knows their part and works together for the greater good. By including family in your recovery plans, you're strengthening your support network and fostering closer relationships built on trust and understanding.

Involving relatives in your postpartum experience can create a tapestry of support that enriches your journey. By communicating openly, setting boundaries, and embracing the unique strengths of each family member, you create an environment where love and assistance flourish. As you continue to build this network, remember that the next chapter will focus on practical coping strategies to support your mental health and well-being. Together, with the help of your loved ones, you can face the challenges ahead with resilience and grace.

CHAPTER 4: PRACTICAL COPING STRATEGIES

Visualize this: you're in the middle of a whirlwind day with your baby, and it feels like the only thing you're juggling is chaos. Between feeding, changing diapers, and trying to remember the last time you brushed your hair, life as a new mom is a dance that often feels more like a clumsy shuffle. But amidst this dance, there's a powerful tool you can wield: mindfulness. It's like a magic wand for your mind, helping you find calm in the storm. Mindfulness isn't about sitting cross-legged on a mountaintop; it's about focusing your attention on the present moment, offering you a lifeline in the sea of motherhood's demands.

Mindfulness, by definition, is the practice of being fully present and engaged with whatever we're doing at the moment—free from distraction or judgment. It's about tuning in to our thoughts and feelings without getting swept away by them. Scientific studies have underscored its benefits, showing that mindfulness can decrease stress-related gray matter in the brain while enhancing areas responsible for memory and creativity.

This is good news for new moms who often feel like their brains are on a permanent vacation. By practicing mindfulness, you can manage stress, increase awareness, and improve emotional regulation, which is a fancy way of saying you'll have fewer meltdowns over spilled milk.

Now, if you're thinking, "Who has time for meditation with a baby in the house?"—you're not alone. Luckily, mindfulness doesn't require hours of solitude. You can practice it in short bursts throughout your day. One of the simplest ways is through breathing exercises. Imagine yourself taking a deep breath in, holding it for a moment, then slowly exhaling, letting go of stress with each breath. This can be done anywhere—while your baby naps or even during those precious seconds of quiet in the shower. Another technique is body scan meditation. This involves mentally scanning your body from head to toe, noticing any tension, and consciously releasing it. It's like a mini-vacation for your mind and body, and no plane ticket is required.

Mindful walking or movement is another way to incorporate mindfulness into your life. Next time you're out with the stroller, focus on the sensation of your feet touching the ground, the sounds around you, or the rhythm of your steps. This transforms an ordinary walk into a grounding experience, helping you reconnect with the present moment.

Mindfulness doesn't just benefit you; it can enhance your interactions with your baby, too. Mindful feeding practices, for instance, involve focusing on the connection between you and your child during mealtimes. Notice their little expressions, the way their tiny hands move. This attention fosters a deeper bond and makes feeding a shared moment of presence. Similarly, engaging fully when playing with your baby, setting aside distractions. Whether it's stacking blocks or making silly faces, being present means you're genuinely sharing in those irreplaceable moments of joy and discovery.

Integrating mindfulness into your daily routine doesn't have to be a chore. Start small by practicing mindful listening during conversations. Give your full attention to the person speaking without planning your next response. It's a practice that not only improves communication but also strengthens relationships.

Practicing gratitude as a daily ritual can also be a powerful mindfulness exercise. Each day, take a moment to reflect on something you're thankful for. It could be as simple as a moment of peace or your baby's infectious giggle. This practice shifts your focus from stress to appreciation, fostering a sense of well-being amid the daily grind.

4.1 Mindfulness Practice Checklist

- Breathing Exercises: Take a few deep breaths, inhaling slowly and exhaling fully. Use this to center yourself during hectic moments.
- Body Scan Meditation: Set aside a few minutes to mentally scan your body, releasing any tension you find.
- Mindful Walking: Focus on your steps and surroundings during your next walk, turning it into a meditative practice.
- Mindful Feeding: Engage fully during feeding times, noticing your baby's responses and connecting deeply.
- Gratitude Ritual: Reflect on one thing you're grateful for each day, enhancing your sense of appreciation and presence.
- Breakfast Smoothie: Blend banana, spinach, almond milk, and peanut butter for a nourishing start.
- One-Pot Dinner: Create a veggie-packed stew with chicken or beans for a comforting meal.
- Hydration Tips: Infuse water with cucumber or lemon, and enjoy herbal teas for variety.

Finding ways to incorporate these foods and practices into your daily routine can do wonders for your mood and energy levels.

Eating well isn't about transforming your life overnight; it's about making small, manageable changes that support your mental and physical health. As you explore these options, remember that taking care of yourself is a vital part of taking care of your family. You deserve to feel your best, and with a few tweaks, you can nurture your body and mind through the power of nutrition.

4.2 Small Steps: Implementing Exercise into Your Routine

Remember the last time you caught a glimpse of your reflection and thought, "Who's that tired superhero?" You're wearing the cape of motherhood, but even superheroes need a boost. Exercise might just be the secret weapon in your arsenal. It's not about chiseling abs or running marathons—unless that's your thing. It's about moving your body and boosting your mood. When you exercise, your body releases endorphins, those magical little chemicals that act as natural mood lifters. They're like nature's Prozac but without the prescription. Regular physical activity can reduce stress and improve sleep quality, helping you feel more energized and balanced. Imagine waking up and not immediately feeling like you've been hit by a freight train. That's the gift of exercise.

You might be thinking, "I barely have time to shower, let alone work out." But here's the thing: exercise doesn't have to be a grand production. Short home workout routines can fit into your schedule like a missing puzzle piece. Think about quick bursts of activity that require minimal equipment, like squats, lunges, or even a few rounds of jumping jacks during nap time. And don't forget about baby-friendly exercises. Stroller walks are perfect for fresh air and bonding time with your little one. It's like multitasking at its finest—you're getting fit while your baby takes in the world. You can also try simple yoga stretches that involve your baby, like gently lifting them while you do a bridge pose. It's a workout and playtime rolled into one.

The hurdles to getting started are real, though. Lack of time and motivation can feel like boulders blocking your path. But setting realistic goals is your bulldozer. Start small, like committing to a ten-minute walk each day. Gradually, you can increase the duration as it becomes a natural part of your routine. Involving your baby in physical activities can also make a world of difference. Babies love movement, and you'll find that a giggling baby makes any workout more fun. Try dancing around the living room with your baby in your arms. It might not look like a traditional workout, but your heart and your baby will thank you.

There's something deeply satisfying about ticking off a goal on your to-do list, and exercise is no exception. Achieving exercise goals can give you a sense of accomplishment, boost your self-esteem, and make you feel like a rockstar mom. Consider tracking your progress with a fitness journal. Write down what you did each day, how you felt afterward, and any milestones you reached. It's a tangible way to see your growth and celebrate your dedication. And speaking of celebrations, don't shy away from them. Maybe you reached a new personal best or completed a week of consistent exercise. Celebrate those victories, no matter how small they seem. Treat yourself to a bath, a new book, or even just a few minutes of peace and quiet.

The beauty of exercise is that it's as much about what it does for your mind as what it does for your body. It's a tool, one that can help you reclaim a little slice of yourself amidst the demands of motherhood. Whether it's a five-minute stretch or a brisk walk around the block, every bit counts, and each step is a win. Embrace these small steps and let them lead you toward a healthier, happier you.

4.3 Managing Sleep Deprivation: Tips for Better Rest

Imagine sleep as a precious commodity, harder to come by than a two-minute shower without interruptions. Sleep deprivation, especially in the postpartum period, can feel like an unwelcome guest that refuses to leave. And it doesn't just affect your ability to function; it can mess with your mind, too. When you're running on empty, your cognitive function takes a nosedive. You might find yourself forgetting where you put the car keys or zoning out mid-conversation. Your mood can also take a hit, swinging from frustration to tears at the drop of a hat. Lack of sleep is like pouring gasoline on the fire of postpartum depression, intensifying feelings of anxiety and overwhelm. It's no wonder that sleep and mental health are so closely linked, each feeding into the other in a cycle that feels hard to break.

But hope is not lost! There are ways to improve sleep quality, even amidst the chaos of new motherhood. Creating a calming bedtime routine can signal to your body that it's time to wind down. Think of it as tucking yourself in with a lullaby for grown-ups. Start by setting a regular sleep schedule, even if it feels impossible with a baby. Consistency can help regulate your internal clock, making it easier to drift off. Consider incorporating soothing activities into your routine, like reading a book or taking a warm bath. These rituals can create a sense of calm, helping your mind and body transition from the hustle of the day to the peace of the night. Power napping is another strategy for squeezing in rest when nighttime sleep is elusive. Short naps of 20-30 minutes can recharge your batteries without leaving you groggy. It's like hitting the reset button on your brain, giving you the energy to face whatever comes your way.

Optimizing your sleep environment can also make a world of difference in the quality of your rest. Reducing noise and light can transform your bedroom into a sanctuary of tranquility. Consider using blackout curtains to keep the room dark and a white noise machine to drown out any disturbances. Comfortable bedding is equally important, like wrapping yourself in a cocoon of coziness. Invest in a good-quality mattress and pillows that support your sleep needs. These small changes can create an environment that encourages restful slumber, making it easier to fall asleep and stay asleep, even if it's just for a couple of hours at a time.

Shared parenting can be a game-changer when it comes to managing sleep with a new baby. Taking turns for night-time feedings can prevent one parent from bearing the brunt of sleep deprivation. Communicating about sleep needs and adjustments is key. Maybe your partner takes the early evening shift while you get a few hours of uninterrupted rest, then you switch roles. It's all about teamwork and finding a rhythm that works for both of you. Open communication ensures that both parents are on the same page and can make necessary adjustments as needed. It's not just about surviving the nights; it's about working together to create a support system that benefits both you and your baby. By sharing the responsibility, you're not just easing the physical burden; you're also fostering a partnership that strengthens your relationship.

4.4 Quick Stress Relievers: Techniques for Immediate Calm

Life as a new mom can sometimes feel like you're navigating a minefield blindfolded while balancing a stack of teetering plates on your head. The unpredictability of each day can send stress levels through the roof, and having quick stress-relief techniques at your fingertips becomes invaluable. These little gems can be utilized in those particularly stressful moments when you feel like you might just lose it. Think of them as your personal toolkit, ready to deploy whenever you need a quick reset. It's about having those effective tools available, like a superhero with gadgets up her sleeve, ready to swoop in and save the day.

One of the simplest yet most effective techniques is deep breathing. It sounds almost too easy, but taking a few deliberate, deep breaths can work wonders. When the baby is fussing, your laundry pile is plotting world domination, and the dishes are auditioning to be Mount Everest, a few deep breaths can help center you. Imagine inhaling calm and exhaling stress. In just a few minutes, you can feel a shift in your energy. Visualization techniques are another powerful ally. Picture yourself in a peaceful place—perhaps a serene beach or a quiet forest. Let your mind wander there for a moment, and you may find your stress melting away, even if just for a few moments. Music and sounds can also provide instant calm. A favorite song or calming nature sounds can transport you to a more peaceful state, offering a much-needed emotional detox.

Having portable stress-relief tools can make all the difference when you're on the go. Stress-relief apps on your smartphone can offer guided meditations, calming music, or even just a few minutes of mindful breathing exercises. They're like carrying a pocket-sized therapist with you, ready to help at a moment's notice. A stress ball or another tactile item can also provide a quick outlet for tension—something to squeeze when words just aren't enough. Keeping these tools handy ensures that you're never without a way to relieve stress, no matter where you are or what chaos is unfolding around you.

Creating your personal stress-relief toolkit is a bit like assembling a first aid kit for your emotions. Start by identifying your personal triggers and responses. Is it the sound of a baby crying that sets you off, or perhaps the sight of a messy house? Recognize what gets your heart racing and your mind spiraling. Once you know your triggers, customize a list of go-to activities that can help calm you down. Maybe it's a favorite breathing exercise, a quick stretch, or even a silly dance with your baby. Having this list ready means you'll know exactly what to do when stress rears its head. It's like having a roadmap to peace, guiding you back to calm whenever you lose your way.

As we wrap up this chapter, it's important to remember that stress is a natural part of life, especially in the whirlwind of motherhood. But with the right tools and techniques, you can navigate these stressful moments with grace and resilience.

Whether it's through quick stress-relief techniques, nourishing your body, or finding moments of calm, you're building a foundation of well-being that supports both you and your family. As we move forward, let's explore how to deepen your connection with your partner, creating a supportive environment that nurtures both your relationship and your role as parents.

CHAPTER 5: NAVIGATING IDENTITY AND EMOTIONS

P icture this: you're at a crowded party, music blaring, people chatting, and there you are, holding a tiny human. Amidst the chaos, you suddenly realize that you're not quite sure who you are anymore. Motherhood has this uncanny ability to turn your identity upside down, leaving you feeling like a stranger in your own life. It's like you've been handed a brand-new script, but no one gave you the lines. This identity shift is a common part of becoming a mom. In fact, it's almost a rite of passage. The transition from being just you to being someone's mother can feel both exhilarating and terrifying. You're still you, but now there's a new role to play, and it's one that demands center stage.

Navigating this transformation requires embracing change and growth in a way that feels authentic to you. One of the most powerful tools at your disposal is journaling. This simple act of putting pen to paper can help you explore the depths of your emotions and gain insight into your evolving identity. Consider starting with prompts like, "What parts of myself do I want to carry forward?" or "What new strengths have I discovered in myself through motherhood?" These reflections can be illuminating, helping you to see the multifaceted person you're becoming. Setting personal growth goals is another way to embrace this change. Whether it's learning a new skill, dedicating time to a hobby, or simply committing to self-care, these goals can serve as beacons, guiding you toward the person you're becoming.

Motherhood doesn't mean putting your interests on hold. In fact, it's an opportunity to explore new passions—or revisit forgotten ones. The key is to find activities that spark joy and curiosity, even in small doses. Joining local or online interest groups can be a great way to connect with like-minded individuals and explore new hobbies. Whether it's a book club, a crafting group, or a virtual cooking class, these gatherings offer a chance to step outside the daily grind and rediscover what excites you. Trying new activities with your baby can also be a fun way to explore new interests. Baby yoga, stroller-friendly hikes, or even baby music classes can become shared experiences that enrich both your lives. It's about finding joy in the everyday and creating new memories together.

Self-reflection and self-compassion are essential companions on this journey. Understanding and accepting the changes you're experiencing can lead to profound personal growth. Practicing daily affirmations can reinforce positive thinking and help you embrace your evolving identity. Try starting each day with simple affirmations like, "I am capable," or "I am worthy of love and happiness." These words might seem small, but they have the power to transform your mindset. Creating a personal mantra for encouragement can also be a powerful tool. It's like having a little cheerleader in your pocket, ready to lift you up whenever you need it. Your mantra could be something as simple as, "I am enough," or as unique as "I am growing and thriving." Whatever resonates with you, let it serve as a gentle reminder that you are doing your best and that you're worthy of grace and kindness.

5.1 Reflection Exercise

Take a moment to write down your thoughts on how motherhood has changed your identity. What aspects of your old self do you miss, and what new qualities do you appreciate? Reflect on how you can integrate these elements into your current life. Use this reflection to create a personal mantra that resonates with your journey.

As you navigate this new normal, remember that you're not alone in these feelings. Countless mothers have walked this path before you, each finding their own way to balance the demands of motherhood with their personal identity. Embrace this chapter of your life with open arms, knowing that every change brings new opportunities for growth and discovery.

5.2 Balancing Roles: Motherhood and Personal Identity

Balancing the roles of motherhood and personal identity might sometimes feel like juggling flaming swords while riding a unicycle. The demands of parenting clash with your personal needs, leaving you wondering if you'll ever have a moment to yourself again. On the one hand, there are diapers to change, meals to prepare, and an endless list of parenting responsibilities that seem to reproduce like rabbits. On the other, there's you, the individual who existed long before the title of "mom" became your calling card. Managing these conflicting demands can be exhausting. Yet, it's essential to remember that you're not just a caretaker; you're a person with dreams, desires, and a unique identity that deserves to thrive alongside your role as a mother.

Prioritizing your personal identity can feel like a radical act in the whirlwind of motherhood, but it's crucial for your well-being. One way to maintain your individuality is by allocating time for personal activities. It might mean setting aside an hour each week for a beloved hobby or sneaking in a chapter of that novel you've been meaning to finish. Establishing boundaries for personal space is equally important. It's okay to claim a corner of your home as your sanctuary, a place where you can retreat for a few moments of peace. Communicate these needs with your family, ensuring they understand the importance of this time for you. It's not about being selfish; it's about nurturing the parts of you that make you whole.

Self-care is often touted as the solution to all of life's woes, but let's be real: it's not always as simple as lighting a candle and taking a bubble bath. True self-care involves actively scheduling personal time for relaxation or hobbies. It might mean waking up a bit earlier for a quiet coffee before the chaos begins or taking a walk during nap time to clear your head. Seeking help with childcare can also facilitate self-care, giving you the opportunity to recharge. Enlist the support of family or friends, or consider hiring a babysitter for a few hours. Remember, caring for yourself ultimately benefits your whole family, as a fulfilled and rested mom is more present and capable of handling parenting challenges.

Integrating your personal and parenting roles can create a harmonious balance that enriches both aspects of your life. One way to do this is by involving your children in your personal interests. If you love painting, let your little one join in with finger paints, turning it into a shared creative experience. If cooking is your passion, invite your kids to help with simple tasks, making meal prep a family affair. Creating family traditions that reflect your personal values can also bridge the gap between self and motherhood. Whether it's a weekly family game night or a monthly nature hike, these traditions can reinforce the values you hold dear while creating lasting memories. It's about blending the personal with the familial, finding joy in the intersection of who you are and the life you've created as a parent.

Balancing these roles isn't a one-size-fits-all endeavor; it's a personal dance that evolves over time. As you navigate the challenges and joys of motherhood, remember that you're not alone in this balancing act. Countless mothers are right there with you, each figuring out their own rhythm. Embrace the chaos, cherish the quiet moments, and know that the effort you put into balancing these roles is a testament to your strength and resilience. You are not just a mother; you are a vibrant, multifaceted individual with a life full of potential.

5.3 Emotional Load: Understanding and Addressing Mental Burdens

Think about this: you're standing in the middle of your living room, surrounded by toys, laundry, and a grocery list that seems to rewrite itself every time you blink. Welcome to the emotional load—the unseen, often unappreciated mental burden that comes with managing a household and family. It's like juggling flaming torches while riding a unicycle, and it's exhausting. Constant decision-making and planning are at the heart of this load. Who's picking up the kids? Did we remember to pay the electricity bill? Is there a snack in the fridge that hasn't yet evolved into a science project? These questions swirl in your mind, adding weight to your already heavy mental backpack. Then there are the invisible tasks—the ones no one sees but somehow always need doing. Replacing the toilet paper roll, remembering birthdays, or keeping track of everyone's shoe sizes. These small tasks accumulate, creating a mental labyrinth that's hard to navigate.

So, how do you lighten this load without losing your sanity? Start by delegating tasks to your partner or family members. It can be as simple as dividing chores or assigning specific responsibilities like meal planning or laundry. This isn't about shirking duties; it's about sharing the load to ensure no one bears the brunt alone. Using organizational tools and apps can also be a lifesaver. A shared family calendar can keep everyone on the same page, reducing the number of times you have to answer, "What's the plan for today?" Task management apps can help you track responsibilities and deadlines, making it easier to distribute tasks evenly. It's like having a personal assistant in your pocket, ready to remind you of what needs doing.

Open communication about emotional burdens is key to managing them effectively. Weekly family meetings can be a great way to discuss what's on everyone's plate and adjust responsibilities as needed. It's a chance to voice concerns, share victories, and ensure that everyone feels heard and supported. Establishing a shared calendar for tasks can also help keep things organized and ensure that nothing falls through the cracks. It's about creating a family culture of teamwork and transparency, where everyone knows what's expected and can step in to help when needed.

Mindfulness and stress-reduction techniques can also play a crucial role in managing emotional load. Mindfulness meditation focused on stress relief can provide a mental reset, helping you approach challenges with a clearer, calmer mind. Consider incorporating time management and prioritization exercises into your routine to help you focus on what truly matters. It's about finding a balance that allows you to breathe, even when life feels overwhelming. Taking a few moments to center yourself can make a world of difference, giving you the resilience to face whatever challenges come your way.

5.4 Handling Overwhelming Guilt: Giving Yourself Grace

There's a silent soundtrack that seems to play on repeat for many mothers, and it's called guilt. It's the feeling that creeps in when you least expect it, whispering that you're not doing enough or that you should be doing more. Maternal guilt is a universal experience fueled by social pressures and unrealistic standards that paint the picture of a perfect mother. Everywhere you look, there are images of moms who have it all together, who bake organic cookies while managing a spotless home and cherubic children. It's easy to fall into the trap of comparing yourself to others, especially in the age of social media, where everyone's highlight reel is on full display. But let's be real: no one has it all figured out. We're all just trying to do our best, one diaper change at a time.

To combat and manage this overwhelming guilt, reframing negative thoughts is a powerful tool. It's about challenging those nagging voices in your head that tell you you're falling short. When the thought "I'm a bad mother" pops up, replace it with something more balanced, like "I'm doing my best, and that's enough." This shift in perspective can lighten the emotional load you carry. Practicing self-forgiveness is equally important. You're going to make mistakes. That's part of being human, not just being a mom. Forgive yourself for those missteps, whether it's forgetting to pack a lunch or snapping at your little one after a long day. Acknowledge the mistake, learn from it, and let it go. Holding onto guilt serves no one, least of all you.

Self-compassion and empathy towards yourself are vital in navigating these feelings. Being kind to yourself isn't just a luxury; it's a necessity. Compassionate self-talk exercises can help cultivate this kindness. Try speaking to yourself as you would a dear friend. Would you tell her she's failing, or would you remind her of all the things she's doing right? Daily gratitude journaling can also foster self-compassion. Each day, jot down a few things you're grateful for, focusing on the small victories and moments of joy that often get overshadowed by guilt. This practice shifts your focus from what's lacking to what's abundant, reminding you of the goodness in your life.

Community support plays a crucial role in overcoming guilt. Sharing your experiences with others can provide immense relief, offering a reminder that you're not alone in this. Parenting support groups can be a sanctuary, a place where you can voice your fears and triumphs without judgment. Whether online or in-person, these groups create connections with other mothers who understand the unique challenges you face. Participating in community discussions can also be healing. Engaging in conversations about motherhood's realities helps dismantle the illusion of perfection and fosters an environment of authenticity and support.

Self-Compassion Exercise

Consider joining a local parenting support group or an online community where you can share your experiences and learn from others. This connection can provide relief from guilt and offer insights into how other mothers navigate similar challenges. Use this opportunity to practice compassionate self-talk, reminding yourself of your strengths and successes.

Remember, you're not in this alone, and together, we can create a culture of acceptance and understanding, where every mother feels seen, heard, and valued.

5.5 The Path to Self-Acceptance: Loving Yourself Fully

Let's take a moment to talk about self-acceptance, that elusive unicorn we often chase but rarely catch. It's a process where you learn to embrace every part of you, the good and the not-so-good. Imagine looking in the mirror and seeing not just the tired eyes and messy hair but also the fierce love and resilience that define your journey through motherhood. Accepting imperfections and vulnerabilities is no small feat; it requires courage to face our flaws without judgment. But doing so opens the door to fulfillment, a sense of peace that comes from knowing you are enough just as you are. Celebrating personal achievements, even the small ones, plays a crucial role here. Whether it's surviving the day on three hours of sleep or getting through a grocery trip with a toddler in tow, these are victories worth acknowledging.

To foster self-love and acceptance, it's helpful to engage in practical activities that boost self-esteem. One such exercise is creating a self-appreciation list. Take some time to write down things you admire about yourself—qualities, accomplishments, moments of kindness. This list serves as a reminder of your strengths, especially on days when doubt creeps in. Another creative way to visualize your goals and dreams is through a vision board. Gather images, quotes, and anything else that inspires you, and arrange them on a board where you can see them daily. It's a tangible representation of where you're headed, a roadmap to your aspirations.

Building a positive self-image is a journey that requires intentional effort. Positive affirmation practices can be a powerful tool in this process. Start each day with affirmations that resonate with you, like "I am strong and capable" or "I am deserving of love and happiness." These affirmations can help shift your mindset, steering it away from self-doubt and toward self-belief. Seeking constructive feedback from trusted friends can also be enlightening. It's not about seeking validation but gaining perspective on how others see the qualities you might overlook. Often, friends can help shine a light on the aspects of yourself that are truly remarkable.

Self-acceptance isn't just about feeling good; it's fundamental to overall well-being. When you love yourself fully, you create a more balanced and happy life. Personal testimonials and success stories often illustrate this beautifully. Many women who have embraced self-acceptance report feeling more at peace, more present, and more joyful in their roles as mothers and individuals. Quotes from mental health experts echo these sentiments, highlighting how self-acceptance fosters resilience and emotional health. It's a reminder that being kind to yourself isn't just beneficial; it's necessary for your mental and emotional health.

As you reflect on these ideas, remember that self-acceptance is an ongoing process. It's filled with ups and downs, but each step forward is a triumph. You are on a path toward embracing all aspects of yourself, learning to love not just the mother you've become but the incredible woman you've always been. This chapter has been about finding that balance and harmony within yourself, a foundation on which you can build a fulfilling life.

As we wrap up this exploration of identity and emotions, let's look forward to the next chapter, where we'll delve into the importance of involving your partner in your postpartum experience. Together, you can navigate the challenges and joys of this transformative time.

CHAPTER 6: INVOLVING YOUR PARTNER

The day my husband and I brought our first son home was nothing short of a circus act. Between juggling diaper changes and trying to remember when we last ate, communication quickly became our lifeline. It was clear that without it, we were two clowns trying to perform a synchronized routine without a script. For any new parent, talking openly and honestly with your partner is crucial. It's the glue that holds your relationship together when life becomes a whirlwind of baby cries and late-night feedings. Open communication helps ensure you're both on the same page and working as a team rather than feeling like you're battling the chaos solo.

Clear and open communication isn't just nice to have; it's necessary to maintain a supportive relationship. It's like having a reliable GPS when navigating the unpredictable terrain of parenthood. But obstacles can arise, like distractions from a crying baby or stress from a long day. Identifying these communication barriers is the first step. Maybe it's about finding the right time to talk when you're both not exhausted or distracted. Scheduling regular conversations can help keep these barriers at bay. Think of it as setting a recurring date with your GPS to recalibrate and ensure you're both heading in the right direction.

When it comes to expressing needs without turning discussions into debates, using "I" statements can be incredibly effective. Instead of saying, "You never help with the baby," try, "I feel overwhelmed when I don't get support." This subtle shift can prevent your partner from getting defensive and keep the conversation productive. Active listening is another critical skill. It's not just about hearing words but truly understanding their meaning. Imagine playing a game of catch, where you toss a ball back and forth rather than bombarding each other with words. Practicing this can enhance understanding and make conversations smoother and more meaningful.

Honesty plays a pivotal role in keeping communication real and authentic. Sharing your emotions and thoughts openly can strengthen your connection and create a safe space for both of you. It's about being vulnerable, even when it feels uncomfortable. Share your fears and vulnerabilities, and set realistic expectations for the support you need. Maybe you're worried about balancing work and home life, or perhaps you're struggling with feelings of inadequacy. By opening up, you invite your partner to do the same, fostering a deeper understanding and a more supportive relationship.

Ongoing dialogue is the backbone of a healthy partnership. Like watering a plant, continuous communication helps your relationship grow and thrive. Daily check-ins or touchpoints can prevent misunderstandings and build trust over time. Whether it's a quick text during the day or a few moments before bed, these interactions keep the lines of communication open. Consider using shared journals or notes as a tool for expressing thoughts and feelings that might be hard to articulate verbally. It's like passing a note in school but with the added benefit of strengthening your bond.

6.1 Communication Exercise: Shared Journals

Start a shared journal with your partner where you can both jot down thoughts, feelings, or concerns. Use it as a tool for reflection and a way to communicate when words are hard to find.

Involving your partner in the postpartum journey is about more than dividing tasks. It's about building a foundation of trust, empathy, and collaboration. By prioritizing honest, open communication, you create a partnership that not only navigates the challenges of early parenthood but thrives amidst them.

6.2 Shared Parenting: Partnering in Parenthood

Contemplate this: you and your partner are like a dynamic duo, ready to tackle the world of parenting with a plan that rivals any superhero team-up. Shared parenting responsibilities are the secret sauce that can transform the chaos of parenthood into a well-oiled machine. By dividing tasks, you not only alleviate stress but also foster a sense of teamwork that strengthens your relationship. It's about creating a shared parenting plan that plays to each partner's strengths and preferences. Maybe one of you is the master of bedtime stories while the other is a wizard with a diaper bag. By identifying these strengths, you can allocate tasks in a way that feels natural and efficient.

To ensure tasks are fairly distributed, it helps to have a system in place. Rotating schedules for childcare and chores can prevent burnout and keep things balanced. One week, you might handle the late-night feedings, and the next, it's your partner's turn. It's like a game of tag, where you're both in tune with each other's rhythms and needs. Digital tools can also be a lifesaver. Shared calendars or apps designed for task management literally keep everyone on the same page. It's like having a virtual assistant that remembers everything so you don't have to. By using these tools, you can track responsibilities and adjust as needed, ensuring that no one feels overwhelmed or overlooked.

Flexibility is the name of the game in shared parenting. Just when you think you've got it all figured out, life throws a curveball, like a teething baby or a sudden work commitment. Being adaptable to accommodate changing needs is crucial. Adjusting roles as circumstances evolve allows you to respond to whatever life throws your way. Maybe this week, you need to step up with more household duties because your partner has a big deadline at work. Or perhaps they take on extra childcare so you can have a much-needed break. Communicating changes in workload or availability keeps resentment at bay and ensures that both partners feel supported and valued.

Collaboration in parenting isn't just beneficial for you and your partner; it has a profound impact on family dynamics. When you work together, you build a unified parenting approach that enhances family harmony. It's like conducting a symphony, where each instrument plays its part to create a beautiful melody. By collaborating, you model teamwork and cooperation for your children, teaching them the importance of working together. This strengthens the family bond, creating an environment where love and support flourish. Your partnership becomes the foundation upon which your family grows, providing stability and security for everyone involved.

Shared Parenting Plan Exercise

Take some time to sit down with your partner and create a shared parenting plan. List out each person's strengths and preferences, and develop a schedule that plays to these. Use a shared calendar or app to track tasks and responsibilities, ensuring that both partners are equally involved in the process.

In shared parenting, the whole is greater than the sum of its parts. By working together, you not only make the load lighter but also enrich the parenting experience. Through collaboration, communication, and flexibility, you create a partnership that supports and uplifts each other, setting the stage for a happy and thriving family life.

6.3 Empathy and Understanding:

Building Emotional Intimacy

Imagine empathy as the bridge between two hearts, a connection that binds you and your partner in a profound understanding of each other's experiences. It's the ability to step into your partner's shoes and feel the world from their perspective, offering a glimpse into their emotions and thoughts. This understanding fosters a deep connection where both partners feel seen and validated. Practicing empathy-building exercises can be transformative. Try this: spend a few minutes each day reflecting on your partner's experiences, considering what challenges they might face and how they perceive the world. This practice can teach you to appreciate their journey and struggles, creating a foundation of respect and compassion.

Reflective listening techniques can further enhance this connection. It's not just about hearing words; it's about truly understanding the message behind them. When your partner shares something, pause and reflect on what you've heard. For example, "It sounds like you're feeling overwhelmed by work right now." This not only shows that you're actively listening but also invites your partner to delve deeper into their feelings. Reflective listening creates a space where both of you can express thoughts freely, knowing they will be met with understanding rather than judgment. It transforms conversations into opportunities for growth, where empathy and connection flourish.

To cultivate emotional intimacy, consider activities that allow you both to share personal stories and experiences. Sometimes, a simple recounting of your day can reveal unexpected insights into each other's lives. Share moments that made you laugh or situations that challenged you. It's through these stories that you build a tapestry of shared experience, weaving together the threads of your lives. Regular emotional check-ins can also deepen your bond. Set aside time to discuss not just the logistics of the day but how you're both feeling emotionally. These check-ins act as a barometer for your relationship, ensuring that you remain attuned to each other's needs and emotions.

Emotional intimacy plays a pivotal role in recovery from postpartum challenges. A strong emotional connection provides a safe space for expressing the complex emotions that accompany this period. When you feel secure in sharing your fears or anxieties, they become less daunting. Your partner's understanding presence can reduce feelings of isolation and loneliness, wrapping you in a comforting blanket of support. This connection can be a lifeline, offering reassurance and stability as you navigate the tumultuous seas of new parenthood. It's about creating a sanctuary where you can both retreat from the world and find solace in each other's arms.

Patience and compassion are the cornerstones of navigating postpartum challenges together. It's vital to acknowledge each other's efforts, recognizing the unseen work that goes into maintaining both the household and your relationship. Celebrate small victories together, whether it's surviving a sleepless night or finding a moment of peace amidst the chaos. These celebrations reinforce your partnership, reminding you both of the strength you possess as a team. Patience allows you to navigate setbacks with grace, understanding that growth is a process, not a destination. Compassion keeps you grounded, offering kindness to both yourself and your partner as you journey through the ups and downs of parenthood.

Building emotional intimacy is not a one-time effort; it's an ongoing process that requires commitment and care. Through empathy, understanding, and shared experiences, you create a relationship that not only supports you both but also thrives on the depth and richness of your connection. It's about finding joy in everyday moments and cherishing the laughter and tears that shape your lives. Together, you can face whatever challenges come your way, knowing that you have each other's backs and hearts.

6.4 Partner's Guide: Supporting Her through PPD

Think of this as a playbook for partners, a guide to being the rock during those shaky times of postpartum depression. Partners have a pivotal role in supporting recovery, acting as both anchors and allies. Recognizing the signs of postpartum depression is the first step. It's not about walking on eggshells but being aware of changes in mood, energy, or behavior. Maybe she's withdrawing from activities she once loved or struggling with persistent sadness. These are cues, not criticisms, and noticing them early can make all the difference.

Once those signs are on the radar, offering practical and emotional support is next. It's about being there, not just in presence but in action. Sometimes, the most loving gesture is a simple one, like preparing a meal or handling household chores. These acts of service can lift the weight of daily tasks, giving her room to breathe and focus on healing. Another way to offer support is by making space for self-care. Encourage her to take breaks, whether it's a walk in the park or an uninterrupted nap. These small windows of respite can be refreshing, like a cool breeze on a hot day, helping her reconnect with herself.

Educating themselves about postpartum depression can be a game changer for partners. Knowledge is power, and understanding what she's going through can foster empathy and patience. Dive into recommended resources on postpartum depression, perhaps a book or article that sheds light on her experience. Attend therapy or support sessions together if she's comfortable with it. It's not about playing therapist but being informed and ready to support her journey. This shared learning experience can strengthen your partnership, showing her she's not in this alone.

Being an advocate means standing by her side, especially when navigating the healthcare system. Accompany her to medical appointments, providing not just a ride but moral support. It's like being her co-pilot, helping to navigate the sometimes overwhelming world of healthcare. Facilitate communication with professionals, ensuring her voice is heard and concerns addressed. This advocacy is not about speaking for her but amplifying her needs, making sure she receives the care and attention she deserves. Through these actions, partners can be a vital part of the healing process, offering a steady hand and a listening ear.

6.5 Activities for Two: Reconnecting as a Couple

When my husband and I first became parents, our world shifted dramatically. Suddenly, our romantic evenings turned into sleep-deprived nights, and our conversations revolved around diaper brands rather than dreamy getaways. But amidst the chaos, we realized that maintaining our connection was crucial. One way we found to reconnect was by planning regular date nights. It didn't have to be anything fancy—a simple dinner at our favorite local spot or a cozy night in with takeout. The key was carving out time just for us. These moments became little pockets of joy, reminding us of the spark that brought us together in the first place. Exploring new hobbies or interests together also added a fresh layer to our relationship. Whether it was trying a dance class or tackling a tricky puzzle, these shared activities infused our routine with excitement and strengthened our bond.

Romance, it turns out, is the glue that holds a partnership together, especially during the whirlwind of early parenthood. Expressing affection through small gestures can be surprisingly powerful. A lingering hug before heading out for the day or a spontaneous kiss while passing each other in the hallway can reignite that romantic flame. And let's not forget the charm of writing love notes or letters. Tucking a sweet note into their bag or leaving a message on the bathroom mirror reminds your partner that they are cherished and adored. These little acts of love can transform ordinary days into extraordinary ones, nurturing a partnership that thrives on affection and connection.

Balancing couple time with parenting duties often feels like a juggling act worthy of a circus. But with a little planning, it's entirely possible to keep those balls in the air. Scheduling a regular couple of times in advance ensures it doesn't get lost in the shuffle of daily life. Treat it like any other important appointment and stick to it. Enlisting help from family or friends for childcare can also create space for you to focus on each other. Imagine the luxury of an uninterrupted evening, knowing your little one is in safe hands. This time away isn't about escapism; it's about returning to each other, refreshed and reconnected.

Shared relaxation and leisure are not just nice-to-haves; they are vital for unwinding and enjoying each other's company. At the end of a long day, there's something magical about curling up together to watch a favorite movie or show. It's a simple pleasure that offers comfort and familiarity, allowing you to relax and enjoy the moment. Going for walks or engaging in outdoor activities can also be incredibly rejuvenating. Whether it's a stroll through the park or a hike on a nearby trail, these moments of shared leisure allow you to reconnect with nature and each other. They provide a break from the hustle, letting you breathe and appreciate the beauty around you.

Building a life together is about more than surviving the demands of parenthood. It's about finding moments of joy and connection amidst the chaos. By prioritizing activities that nurture your relationship, you create a foundation of love and support that sustains you both. As you continue this journey, remember that these moments are the glue that holds you together, enriching your lives and deepening your bond. They are the quiet strength that carries you through, reminding you of the love that started it all.

CHAPTER 7: DIVERSE PERSPECTIVES AND INCLUSIVE PRACTICES

I magine that you're seated at a family gathering, a warm cup of tea in hand, surrounded by relatives recounting tales of their own parenting escapades. Each story has its own cultural flavor, a mix of customs and traditions that have been passed down through generations. This tapestry of cultural narratives shapes how we view motherhood and the postpartum period. It's a reminder that while we may all be mothers, the journey can be as varied as the spices in a well-stocked pantry.

Cultural beliefs play a major role in shaping postpartum experiences. In many cultures, traditional practices like postpartum confinement are designed to offer new mothers rest and support. Take "doing the month" in Chinese culture, for instance. This practice involves a 30-day period where the new mother rests and is cared for by family, with an emphasis on nourishing foods and avoiding colds. Sounds like a dream, right? Studies suggest that these traditions can alleviate postpartum depression symptoms by providing much-needed social support and rest (SOURCE 1). However, not all cultural practices offer such solace. In some places, cultural beliefs may contribute to postpartum challenges, such as when gender biases or expectations weigh heavily on a new mother.

Then there's the elephant in the room: the cultural stigma surrounding mental health. In some cultures, discussing mental health is as taboo as discussing politics at a family dinner. The fear of judgment and the desire to "save face" can prevent mothers from seeking the help they need. This stigma is not only isolating but can delay treatment, potentially leading to more severe health complications (SOURCE 2). You might feel pressure to appear as the perfect mother, holding everything together when, in reality, you're barely keeping your head above water. Recognizing and challenging these stigmas is crucial for creating an environment where seeking help is seen as a sign of strength, not weakness.

Family support structures also vary widely across cultures. In some traditions, multigenerational households are the norm, providing built-in support for new mothers. Grandparents, aunts, and uncles often play active roles in childcare, allowing mothers to recuperate and adjust to their new roles. In contrast, other cultures may emphasize maternal independence, where the mother is expected to handle responsibilities on her own. These expectations can shape the postpartum experience significantly. On one hand, a robust family network can lighten the load and offer emotional support. On the other, the pressure to fulfill traditional maternal roles can feel overwhelming, especially if they clash with modern lifestyles.

7.1 Reflection Exercise: Exploring Cultural Influences on Your Postpartum Experience

Take a moment to reflect on how your cultural background has influenced your postpartum experience. Consider the traditions and expectations you've encountered. How have they shaped your view of motherhood? What cultural practices have been supportive, and which have been challenging? Write down your thoughts and feelings, and consider sharing them with a trusted friend or support group.

Cultural identity also plays a significant role in shaping self-perception and mental health. Balancing traditional and modern identities can feel like walking a tightrope. You may feel torn between adhering to cultural expectations and embracing contemporary norms. This balancing act can impact your self-esteem and mental health as you navigate the pressures of cultural conformity while striving to assert your individuality. Coping with cultural pressures requires resilience and self-awareness as you seek to honor your heritage while carving out your own path.

Understanding the diverse cultural influences on postpartum experiences can foster empathy and inclusion. It reminds us that there is no one-size-fits-all approach to motherhood and that each journey is as unique as the individual navigating it. By acknowledging and embracing these differences, we create a richer tapestry of support that celebrates the beauty of diversity.

7.2 Stories from Around the World: Diverse Experiences of PPD

In a small village in rural India, Rekha sat on the edge of her woven cot, staring at the vibrant colors of her sari, a stark contrast to the gray cloud of emotions hovering over her. The birth of her child was supposed to be a time of celebration, a joyful addition to her family. But instead of rejoicing, Rekha felt trapped in a cycle of sadness and fatigue. In her community, mental health wasn't something openly discussed, as if acknowledging it would invite shame upon the family. Yet, Rekha found solace in the company of women at the local well. There, amidst the rhythmic sounds of water and laughter, she discovered a network of support. The women shared stories, whispered secrets of herbal remedies, and offered shoulders to lean on. It was in these moments of shared vulnerability that Rekha began to see a glimmer of hope.

Across the globe, in the bustling streets of Tokyo, Yuki navigated the demands of urban life with a newborn in tow. Her apartment felt like an island amidst a sea of skyscrapers, isolating her from the vibrant city she once loved. The pressure to be the perfect mother weighed heavily on her, exacerbated by the unspoken expectation to seamlessly balance work and family life. Yuki found herself lost in a culture that emphasized endurance and self-reliance. However, a chance encounter with a community group dedicated to new mothers changed her perspective. Surrounded by women who echoed her struggles, Yuki learned to embrace the concept of "amae," the Japanese idea of relying on others. The group became her sanctuary, a place where shared experiences transformed isolation into connection.

Meanwhile, in the suburbs of the U.S., Maria, a first-generation immigrant, grappled with the challenges of postpartum depression in a country that sometimes felt foreign and unwelcoming. The layered complexities of cultural identity and motherhood made her feel like she was constantly straddling two worlds. Maria's journey was marked by a longing for familiarity with her home country and the burden of raising a child in a new culture. Yet, she found strength in the multicultural tapestry of her local community center. Here, Maria connected with other immigrant mothers, each with their own tales of triumph and hardship. Together, they formed a vibrant support network, weaving their diverse backgrounds into a rich mosaic of understanding and empathy.

Despite the geographical and cultural differences, there are universal threads that connect experiences of postpartum depression across the globe. Feelings of isolation and loneliness are common, whether you're in a bustling metropolis or a quiet village. The struggle with identity and self-worth is another shared challenge as new mothers navigate the uncharted waters of parenthood while grappling with societal expectations. These experiences remind us that, regardless of where we are, the emotional landscape of postpartum depression often echoes the same notes of vulnerability and resilience.

Cultural practices can offer unique strengths in managing postpartum depression. Community-based support systems, like the women at the well in Rekha's village, provide an invaluable sense of belonging and solidarity. These networks create spaces where women can share their fears without judgment, drawing strength from one another. Traditional healing practices and remedies passed down through generations also play a crucial role in supporting mental health. Herbal teas, meditation, and rituals are woven into the fabric of many cultures, offering comfort and healing. They remind us that the wisdom of our ancestors can be a source of solace.

Lessons learned from diverse perspectives highlight the importance of integrating modern medicine with traditional practices. In Yuki's support group, the combination of contemporary therapeutic approaches and cultural concepts like "amae" created a holistic framework for healing. This blend of old and new underscores the value of adaptability and openness. Building cross-cultural support networks, as seen in Maria's community center, fosters an environment where diverse approaches to postpartum care can flourish. These networks encourage the exchange of ideas, enriching our understanding of postpartum depression and empowering mothers to seek the support they need.

In sharing these stories from around the world, we embrace the diversity of postpartum experiences and celebrate the resilience of mothers everywhere. We acknowledge that while each journey is unique, the bonds of empathy and understanding transcend cultural boundaries, illuminating a path toward healing for all.

7.3 Culturally Sensitive Support: Tailoring Help to Fit You

Imagine walking into a therapist's office, your heart pounding with the weight of the world, hoping they'll understand the tangled mess of emotions you're carrying. You sit down, and within moments, you realize they have no clue about your cultural background, the nuances that make your experience unique. It's like trying to explain the plot of a foreign film without subtitles. This is where culturally sensitive mental health care becomes crucial. It's about ensuring that healthcare providers are not just aware of cultural differences but genuinely understand them. Cultural competence means they've taken the time to learn about different traditions, beliefs, and values that influence mental health. They acknowledge that what works for one person might not work for another, and they respect those differences by creating personalized care plans that align with your cultural preferences. It's like tailoring a suit; it needs to fit you perfectly, not just be pulled off the rack.

Finding culturally sensitive support can feel like searching for a needle in a haystack, but there are strategies to make the process smoother. Start by seeking out directories that list culturally competent therapists. These directories often provide detailed profiles so you can find someone who resonates with your needs. Community resources and cultural organizations can also be invaluable. They often have connections with practitioners who understand the cultural landscape you're navigating. Whether it's a local cultural center or an online forum, these resources can guide you to the support that feels right. It's about creating a network of care that respects and honors your cultural identity.

Language and communication can be formidable barriers to accessing mental health care. Imagine pouring your heart out, only to realize that the person on the other end doesn't understand your words or their meaning fully. Language differences can impact the effectiveness of therapy and lead to misunderstandings. This is where translation services come into play. They can bridge the gap, ensuring that your voice is heard and your needs are understood. But it's not just about translating words; it's about conveying the emotions and subtleties that make your story yours. Clear communication in therapy is vital, as it fosters trust and ensures that you and your provider are on the same page. It's like tuning a radio to the right frequency; without clarity, the message gets lost in static.

Self-advocacy is your superpower when it comes to seeking culturally appropriate care. Don't be afraid to speak up for your needs and preferences. Before meeting with a healthcare provider, prepare questions related to cultural considerations. Ask about their experience with patients from similar backgrounds and discuss how they incorporate cultural elements into their practice. This conversation can set the tone for a therapeutic relationship built on mutual respect and understanding. Communicating your cultural needs to providers might feel daunting, but remember, you're the expert on your own experience. Assert your preferences, whether it's incorporating traditional practices or addressing specific cultural challenges. Your voice matters, and it's your right to ensure that the care you receive reflects who you are.

As we navigate the complex world of postpartum depression, it's essential to remember that culturally sensitive support isn't just a nice-to-have; it's a necessity. It's about creating a space where you feel seen, heard, and valued, where your cultural identity is not a footnote but a central part of your care. So, as you seek support, hold onto the knowledge that you deserve a tailored approach, one that honors the rich tapestry of your life experiences. You're not alone in this, and there's a world of support waiting to embrace you exactly as you are.

7.4 The Power of Stories: Finding Solace in Shared Narratives

Imagine sitting around a cozy campfire with friends, the flames casting dancing shadows, and the night air filled with the sound of shared laughter and whispered secrets. This setting is akin to the comfort and connection storytelling can bring, especially for mothers navigating the choppy waters of postpartum depression. Sharing personal stories has a remarkable therapeutic value. It's like airing out a stuffed closet, allowing fresh air and light to touch places that have been hidden away. When you tell your story, you not only release the burden of carrying it alone, but you also invite others to find solace in the shared experience. Storytelling becomes a tool for healing and connection, a bridge linking you to others who have walked similar paths. It's about finding common ground, where empathy and understanding can flourish, softening the edges of isolation.

Participating in storytelling groups or forums can be a powerful way to engage with this process. Think of these spaces as modern-day campfires, where mothers gather to share and listen. Storytelling workshops offer structured environments where you can hone your narrative, guided by facilitators who create a safe space for expression. These workshops invite you to explore your experiences, encouraging reflection and growth. Online narrative communities offer another avenue, allowing you to connect with others from the comfort of your home. In these virtual spaces, you can share your story with a supportive audience, gaining insights from those who resonate with your words. The act of sharing in these groups transforms your story from a solitary experience into a communal one, deepening connections and fostering a sense of belonging.

Stories hold immense power in reducing stigma. Personal narratives can challenge stereotypes and misconceptions about postpartum depression, illuminating truths that might otherwise remain hidden. When you share your story, you contribute to a larger tapestry of voices that collectively debunk myths and reshape cultural perceptions. Public storytelling, whether through written articles, podcasts, or spoken word events, can shift the narrative around mental health. These stories challenge the notion that postpartum depression is a sign of weakness or failure. They highlight the strength and resilience required to navigate such challenges, offering a counter-narrative that promotes understanding and empathy. By sharing your experience, you become an advocate for change, paving the way for others to do the same.

Crafting and sharing your personal story might feel daunting, but it's a process worth embracing. Start by structuring your narrative, focusing on key moments that define your experience. Consider the emotions and insights that emerged during your journey, and let them guide your storytelling. Think of your story as a tapestry woven with threads of vulnerability and strength. Using storytelling as a tool for advocacy allows you to not only share your journey but also inspire others to seek help and embrace their own narratives. It's about creating a ripple effect, where each story shared encourages another to step into the light. As you craft your story, remember that it's uniquely yours, and its power lies in its authenticity.

The act of storytelling is a gift, both to yourself and to those who hear it. It's an opportunity to transform your experience into something meaningful, a testament to your resilience and courage. By sharing your story, you contribute to a collective narrative that empowers mothers everywhere. You become part of a movement that challenges stigma, fosters connection, and promotes healing. So gather your courage, find your voice, and let your story be heard. You never know who might be listening and how your words might touch their heart.

As we wrap up this chapter on diverse perspectives and inclusive practices, it's clear that embracing our stories, cultures, and identities enriches our understanding of postpartum experiences. Next, we will explore how professional insights and resources can further support your postpartum journey, providing the tools and guidance needed to navigate this transformative time. Together, we continue to build a supportive community, one story at a time.

CHAPTER 8: PROFESSIONAL INSIGHTS AND RESOURCES

Y ou know how when you buy an appliance, it comes with a manual full of helpful tips and tricks? If only babies came with those! Instead, we have experts—real-life superheroes armed with years of study and experience—ready to guide us through the labyrinth of postpartum depression. Let's dive into what these professionals have to say because if there's one thing we all need, it's a little expert advice that doesn't involve deciphering hieroglyphics.

8.1 Insights from the Experts: What Professionals Say About PPD

Mental health experts have spent decades untangling the complex web of postpartum depression. Their insights are like a lifeline thrown to us in the choppy sea of new motherhood. According to leading psychiatrists and psychologists, postpartum depression is not just a phase. Dr. Samantha Meltzer-Brody, a prominent figure in this field, emphasizes that PPD is a genuine medical condition that requires attention, not a reflection of inadequate parenting. She states, "Postpartum depression is a real illness, and like any illness, it needs appropriate treatment and care." Understanding this from the outset can help lift the weight of self-blame that so many mothers carry.

Recent research has illuminated the hormonal and environmental factors contributing to PPD. These studies show that the dramatic shifts in hormones post-birth can act like a spark in a powder keg of emotional and physical changes. The UNC School of Medicine recently conducted a groundbreaking genomic study revealing that about 14% of PPD cases can be attributed to genetic factors (SOURCE 1). It's not just hormones and sleepless nights; there's a biological component, too. Recognizing the genetic links to PPD can be a game-changer for many mothers, offering a new perspective on why they feel the way they do.

Experts are also keen to debunk common myths surrounding PPD. For instance, there's a misconception that postpartum depression always presents immediately after childbirth. In truth, symptoms can develop anytime within the first year. It's like a surprise party you didn't want, showing up when you're least prepared. Another myth is that PPD only affects mothers who've had difficult pregnancies or births. Experts clarify that even those with picture-perfect pregnancies can experience PPD. The key takeaway? PPD doesn't discriminate.

The importance of professional intervention cannot be overstated. Early detection and intervention can make a world of difference. Dr. Patrick Sullivan, a leading researcher, advocates for comprehensive treatment plans tailored to each individual's needs. He explains, "A one-size-fits-all approach doesn't work with PPD. Each mother's experience is unique, and so should be her treatment." Early intervention can prevent the condition from escalating, much like putting out a small fire before it spreads. This can include therapy, medication, and lifestyle adjustments, all coordinated by healthcare professionals who understand the intricacies of PPD.

In the realm of research and treatment, exciting developments are on the horizon. New therapeutic approaches are currently under study and promise to expand the options available to mothers. Advances in personalized medicine and genetics are paving the way for treatments tailored to each individual's genetic makeup. Imagine a world where treatment is as unique as your fingerprint, designed to address your specific needs. This personalized approach could revolutionize how postpartum depression is managed, offering hope to mothers everywhere.

Reflection Exercise

Take a moment to jot down any myths about postpartum depression you've encountered. How have these myths influenced your perception of PPD or your willingness to seek help? Reflect on how understanding the truths shared by experts can empower you to take informed steps toward managing your mental health.

Professionals in the field of mental health provide invaluable insights and guidance for those navigating postpartum depression. Their research and expertise offer a beacon of hope, illuminating the path to recovery with compassion and understanding. By tapping into their knowledge, you're not just arming yourself with information; you're building a support system that extends beyond your immediate circle. These experts are your allies, ready to guide you through the complexities of postpartum depression with empathy and precision.

8.2 Therapy and Counseling: What to Expect

Therapy can feel like stepping into a new world, one where you finally get to untangle the messy ball of yarn that's been on your mind lately. It's like having a guide who helps you navigate the twists and turns of postpartum depression with a roadmap tailored just for you. There are several types of therapy available, each offering something unique. Cognitive Behavioral Therapy (CBT) is one of the most commonly recommended therapies. It's like having a personal trainer for your brain, helping you reframe negative thought patterns into positive ones. Imagine transforming that nagging voice that says, "I'm not good enough," into, "I'm doing the best I can, and that's enough." CBT empowers you to take control of those spiraling thoughts and replace them with healthier narratives.

Interpersonal Therapy (IPT) focuses on the relationships and social dynamics that surround you. It's like having a heart-to-heart with your best friend but with someone who's trained to help you navigate complex social landscapes. Whether it's managing the shifting dynamics with your partner or addressing role transitions, IPT offers tools to enhance your interpersonal toolkit. It's especially beneficial if you feel like your relationships have taken a hit since the baby arrived. Then there's group therapy, which can be incredibly validating. Imagine sitting in a circle with other moms who get it, sharing experiences and supporting each other. It's like finding your tribe, where you can be open and honest without fear of judgment.

The therapy process often begins with an initial assessment. Think about this like the first chapter in a book, where you set the scene and outline the plot. It's a chance for you and your therapist to get to know each other and establish what you hope to achieve. This session might involve discussing your symptoms, your history, and any specific goals you have in mind. From there, you'll work together to create a treatment plan tailored to your needs. Sessions are typically held once a week, although this can vary depending on your situation. Each session builds on the last, like adding layers to a lasagna until you've got a rich, flavorful dish. Homework assignments might be part of the process, but don't worry; these aren't like traditional school assignments. They're more like practical exercises designed to reinforce what you've learned in therapy. Think of them as little steps that help you track your progress and keep you moving forward.

The therapist-client relationship is a cornerstone of effective therapy. It's crucial to find someone you feel comfortable with, like finding the perfect pair of jeans that fit just right. Building trust and rapport takes time, but it's worth the effort. This relationship is a partnership where open communication is key. Don't be afraid to express your preferences and concerns. If something isn't working for you, it's okay to speak up. Your therapist is there to support you, not to judge you. This is your space to explore your thoughts and feelings openly, without fear of judgment. It's about creating an environment where you feel safe and heard, like a cozy corner where you can just be yourself.

Concerns about therapy are common, and it's natural to have questions about what to expect. Confidentiality and privacy are paramount, akin to the therapist-client relationship being akin to a vault where your secrets are kept safe. Everything you share in therapy stays there, providing a secure space to explore your thoughts and feelings. You might also worry about facing emotional challenges during sessions. Therapy can be tough, like peeling back layers of an onion, but it's also an opportunity for growth and healing. Your therapist is trained to guide you through this process with compassion and understanding. They'll help you navigate any emotional turbulence, offering support and reassurance along the way. Remember, reaching out for help isn't a sign of weakness; it's a testament to your strength and determination to feel better.

8.3 Resources at Your Fingertips: Books, Apps, and More

Navigating the waters of postpartum depression can feel like being adrift at sea. Sometimes, you need a guiding light to show you the way. Books have always been my go-to for comfort and wisdom, and there's a treasure trove out there dedicated to postpartum depression. These books are like having a seasoned friend by your side, offering both solace and practical advice. Titles like "Down Came the Rain" by Brooke Shields provide personal stories that resonate deeply, reminding you that even celebrities aren't immune to these struggles. If you're yearning for expert advice, "This Isn't What I Expected" by Karen Kleiman and Valerie Raskin dives into coping strategies and exercises designed to help you regain control. These books aren't just pages and ink; they're voices of experience ready to guide you through the fog with both empathy and expertise.

But let's not forget the digital age we live in. There are mental health apps designed to be your pocket-sized therapist. Apps like "MoodTools" help you track your feelings and identify patterns over time. It's like having a little notebook that keeps tabs on your emotional well-being without any judgment. If you're feeling frazzled, "Headspace" offers guided meditation to help calm the chaos inside your mind. Imagine a soothing voice guiding you to a place of peace, even if it's just for a few minutes a day. These apps are more than just digital tools; they're companions that remind you to breathe, pause, and take a moment for yourself amid the whirlwind of motherhood.

In the quest for understanding and skill-building, online courses and workshops offer a wealth of knowledge. Parenting workshops with a mental health focus are like attending a class where the syllabus is all about you and your needs as a new mom. Webinars led by mental health professionals provide insights that can be transformative. Picture a virtual classroom where you're surrounded by other parents, all eager to learn and support each other. These courses are more than just educational; they're communities of learning and growth, offering the chance to connect with others and gain valuable skills in a supportive environment.

When you feel like you're at the end of your rope, knowing where to turn for immediate support can be a lifesaver. A directory of support organizations and hotlines should be on your fridge, ready to grab when needed. Organizations like Postpartum Support International offer resources and support groups tailored specifically for new mothers. They're like a lifeline reaching out to you, ready to pull you back to safety. Crisis hotlines provide immediate assistance when you need someone to talk to, ensuring that you're never truly alone. These resources are the safety nets designed to catch you when you feel like you're falling, providing a foundation of support that can make all the difference.

Resource List

Here's a handy list of resources:

- Books: "Down Came the Rain" by Brooke Shields, "This Isn't What I Expected" by Karen Kleiman and Valerie Raskin
- Apps: MoodTools, Headspace
- Courses/Workshops: Online parenting workshops with a mental health focus, webinars from health professionals
- Support: Postpartum Support International, crisis hotlines

Navigating postpartum depression can feel overwhelming, but you have an arsenal of resources at your disposal. Whether it's the comforting words of a book, the guidance of an app, the knowledge from a webinar, or the support from a hotline, these tools are here to help. They're not just resources; they're your allies, ready to assist whenever you need a helping hand.

8.4 Navigating the Healthcare System: Accessing the Right Care

Finding the right healthcare provider for postpartum depression can Feel like hunting for a needle in a haystack that keeps shifting in the wind. It's about fit and comfort, and sometimes, it involves trying on a few before settling on the right one. Start by researching provider credentials and specialties. You want someone who's not just a therapist but a specialist in postpartum depression. It's akin to choosing a chef who specializes in your favorite cuisine. Look for mental health professionals with experience and training in perinatal mental health. Understanding the different types of professionals can also help you make an informed decision. Psychiatrists can prescribe medication and are often invaluable when medication is part of the treatment plan. Psychologists and social workers, meanwhile, offer therapeutic support and can be instrumental in helping you work through emotional challenges. The key is to find someone who speaks your language—both literally and figuratively.

Navigating the insurance landscape is like weaving through a maze. It's not always clear, and the paths can be winding. Start by checking your insurance policy to see what's covered. Some plans offer extensive mental health benefits, while others may have limitations. Understanding these details can save you from unpleasant surprises down the line. If your insurance falls short, financial assistance options might be available. Sliding scale fees, which adjust based on your income, can make therapy more affordable. Community mental health centers often provide services at reduced rates. It's a bit like finding a hidden gem in a thrift store; sometimes, a little digging can reveal treasures that fit your needs perfectly.

Being an advocate for yourself within the healthcare system is crucial. Picture yourself as the captain of your own ship, steering through the waters of healthcare with confidence. Prepare for appointments by jotting down questions and concerns. This preparation turns what could be a daunting experience into a structured dialogue. Be clear about your needs and preferences when speaking with providers. It's your health on the line, and your voice matters. If something doesn't feel right, don't hesitate to speak up. You're not just a patient; you're an active participant in your care. And remember, it's okay to shop around until you find a provider who meets your expectations and makes you feel supported.

Coordinated care is like an orchestra, with each instrument playing its part. Your primary care physician, therapist, and any specialists need to be in harmony, working together to support your well-being. This collaboration ensures that you receive comprehensive care. Your primary care physician can be a valuable ally, offering referrals to specialists and coordinating your overall treatment plan. Don't hesitate to ask for referrals if you feel that specialized care is needed. It's a bit like assembling a team of experts, each bringing their unique talents to the table. When everyone is on the same page, you benefit from a seamless, integrated approach that addresses all aspects of your health.

Navigating the healthcare system can be daunting, but with the right tools and mindset, you can find the support you need. Think of it as building a support network where each provider plays a vital role in your recovery. As you navigate this path, remember that you're not alone. There's a community of professionals ready to support you, with each step bringing you closer to the care you deserve. With the right guidance and persistence, you can access the resources and support necessary to manage postpartum depression effectively.

In the next chapter, we'll delve into interactive and reflective practices, exploring ways to engage with your emotions and track your progress toward healing. These practices will offer tangible steps to complement the professional care you receive, empowering you to reclaim your well-being and embrace the journey ahead.

CHAPTER 9: INTERACTIVE AND REFLECTIVE PRACTICES

I magine standing on the edge of a bridge, tossing a pebble into the water below. The ripples spread outward, touching every part of the pond. This simple act of release can be remarkably similar to the experience of journaling, where each word you write sends ripples through your mind and heart, offering clarity and understanding. Journaling can be an invaluable tool, especially during the postpartum period when emotions are as unpredictable as a toddler with a permanent marker. It's a form of self-care that provides a safe space to explore the messy, beautiful chaos of new motherhood.

Through the act of writing, you allow thoughts and feelings to flow onto the page without judgment or reservation. This cathartic process can bring a sense of relief, like opening a window to let in fresh air. When you journal regularly, you create a dialogue with yourself, leading to improved mental clarity and emotional processing. It's not about crafting perfect prose. Instead, imagine it as a conversation with a dear friend, where honesty and vulnerability are encouraged. Regular journaling can help untangle the knotted emotions that often accompany postpartum depression, giving you a clearer view of your inner landscape.

To get started, consider some journaling prompts tailored to postpartum experiences. Reflecting on daily emotions and experiences can be as simple as jotting down what made you smile today or what felt like an insurmountable challenge. Explore your fears and hopes related to motherhood. What are you most afraid of? What dreams do you hold for yourself and your child? Writing letters to yourself or your baby can also be powerful. Imagine penning a letter to your future self or capturing a moment you want your baby to remember. These prompts encourage introspection and emotional exploration, offering insights into your journey.

Experimenting with different journaling methods can help you find what resonates most with you. If you prefer concise entries, bullet journaling might be your style. It allows for quick reflections, perfect for those days when time is short, and the baby is particularly demanding. Alternatively, dialogue journaling can be a way to explore internal conflicts. Picture it as a conversation between different parts of yourself, where you can express worries, offer reassurance, and find a resolution. These varied formats cater to different preferences and needs, ensuring that journaling becomes a personalized practice that supports your mental health.

Incorporating journaling into your daily routine can transform it from an occasional activity into a habit that nurtures your well-being. Start by setting aside dedicated journaling time, perhaps during your morning coffee or before settling into bed. This consistent practice can turn journaling into a ritual, providing a moment of calm in your day. Creating a comfortable journaling space can also enhance the experience. Find a cozy nook, light a candle, or play soft music. These small touches can invite relaxation and creativity, making journaling a cherished part of your routine.

9.1 Journaling Prompts

Here are some prompts to help you get started:

- What emotions have surfaced today?
- Reflect on a moment of joy or challenge.
- What are your hopes for tomorrow?
- Write a letter to your baby about what you love most about them.
- What would you like your future self to remember about this time?

As you embrace journaling, remember that there's no right or wrong way to do it. It's a practice tailored to your needs and experiences, offering a space for reflection and healing. Whether you write a few lines or fill pages with thoughts, each entry is a step toward understanding yourself more deeply. Let the words flow, trusting that they'll guide you to greater clarity and peace.

9.2 Progress Tracking: Celebrating Small Wins

Remember the first time your baby smiled, that tiny curl of lips that seemed to light up the entire room? Just like that smile, the small wins in your recovery deserve to be cherished and celebrated. Monitoring your progress through postpartum depression can be like keeping a record of these little victories. It's about recognizing the days when you felt the weight lift just a bit or when you managed to find a moment of peace amidst the chaos. Tracking progress isn't just about the end goal; it's about acknowledging the journey you're on and every step you take along the way. When you see your improvements laid out before you, it's easier to understand that change is happening, even if it's incremental. This awareness can be a powerful motivational tool, like a little nudge that says, "You've got this. Keep going."

One way to keep an eye on your progress is by creating a visual progress chart. Think of it as your personal map, charting the highs, lows, and everything in between. It could be as simple as a calendar where you jot down a word or a color that represents your mood each day. Over time, you'll have a visual representation of your journey, a tapestry woven with the threads of your experiences. If you're more digitally inclined, there are plenty of apps designed for mood and activity tracking. These apps can offer insights into patterns you might not notice otherwise. They're like a pocket-sized therapist, gently reminding you of how far you've come. Whether you choose a chart or an app, the key is consistency. Regular updates create a clearer picture of your growth.

Celebrating small victories is another essential part of progress tracking. It's like throwing confetti for yourself every time you hit a milestone, no matter how small. Maybe you finally had the courage to attend a support group, or perhaps you managed a full night's sleep without waking up in a panic. These wins deserve recognition. Consider planning small rewards for yourself when you reach these milestones. It doesn't have to be extravagant —a favorite snack, a bubble bath, or a new book can be a meaningful acknowledgment of your progress. Sharing these successes with a support network can amplify the joy. When you tell a friend or a loved one about your achievements, you're not only celebrating but also strengthening the bonds of connection. Their encouragement can be a balm, reinforcing your efforts and reminding you that you're supported.

Reflection plays a significant role in recognizing how far you've come. It's about looking back with compassion and understanding, like flipping through a photo album and appreciating each snapshot of your life. Reflective journaling on achievements allows you to capture these moments in words, to see the growth and transformation you might otherwise overlook. Reviewing past entries can be enlightening. You might find that what once seemed insurmountable now feels like a distant memory. These reflections can serve as beacons of hope, guiding you through rough patches and reminding you of your resilience. They're a testament to your strength, a collection of proof that you are capable of overcoming challenges and emerging stronger on the other side.

9.3 Reflective Questions: Deepening Your Understanding

Have you ever found yourself standing in front of the fridge, door wide open, and wondering, "What am I even doing here?" Sometimes, life feels like that. Especially when you're knee-deep in motherhood, trying to keep your head above water. That's where reflective questions can come into play. They act like a compass, helping you navigate the swirling sea of emotions and responsibilities. Asking yourself questions like, "What are my current emotional needs?" can feel like shining a flashlight into the dark corners of your mind. It's about pinpointing what you truly need in this moment, whether it's a hug, a nap, or just a good cry. And don't underestimate the power of asking, "How have my priorities changed since becoming a parent?" It might surprise you to see how your values have shifted, how the little things you once stressed over now pale in comparison to your child's giggle. Or perhaps, "In what ways can I practice more self-compassion?" is the question that resonates with you, urging you to treat yourself with the same kindness you offer a friend. These questions aren't just queries—they're invitations to explore deeper layers of your being.

Reflective questioning isn't just about asking the right questions, though. It's about unlocking a door to personal growth. They encourage you to put on your thinking cap and dig deeper, beyond the surface-level worries of diaper changes and bedtime routines. When you engage in critical thinking and self-analysis, you start to identify patterns in your thoughts and behaviors. Maybe you notice that every time the laundry piles up, so does your anxiety. Or perhaps you realize that your habit of staying up late to watch Netflix is your way of carving out "me time." These insights can be the catalysts for change, leading to breakthroughs that shift how you approach the challenges of motherhood. They're like little light bulbs going off in your mind, illuminating new paths to explore.

Answering reflective questions requires more than just a casual thought. It's about diving in and truly exploring your responses. Free writing is a fantastic technique for this. Set a timer, grab a notebook, and let your thoughts flow without judgment. Don't worry about grammar or coherence—just write. It's like having a conversation with yourself, where no one's there to interrupt or critique. If writing isn't your thing, try discussing these questions with a trusted confidant. Sometimes, verbalizing your thoughts to someone else can offer new perspectives and insights. They might ask a follow-up question that takes your reflection in an unexpected direction, opening up new areas for contemplation.

Regular reflection is like watering a plant; it nurtures continuous growth. By setting regular times for reflection, you're creating a habit that fosters long-term development. Maybe it's during your morning coffee or perhaps at night once everyone's asleep. Routine reflection can become a ritual that anchors your day, providing moments of clarity amidst the chaos. Incorporating reflection into daily routines doesn't have to be monumental. It can be as simple as spending five minutes in the shower thinking about something that challenged you today or mentally noting what brought you joy. These small acts of introspection accumulate, like drops filling a bucket, leading to significant growth over time.

Reflection Exercise

Here's a simple exercise to help guide your reflection: Choose one question each day and spend five minutes exploring it. You might write your thoughts, talk them out, or simply ponder them during a quiet moment. Notice any patterns or insights that emerge, and consider how they influence your daily life and decisions. This practice isn't about perfection; it's about progress and understanding.

9.4 Creative Outlets: Expressing Yourself Through Art

When words seem to fail us, art steps in, offering an alternative language of colors, textures, and shapes. Creative activities can be like taking a deep breath after holding it for too long, allowing emotions to flow freely without the need for structured sentences or perfect grammar. Imagine standing before a blank canvas, brush in hand, ready to spill your heart onto it. There's something deeply therapeutic about this process. Art becomes a vessel for emotions, a non-verbal way to communicate what might be too complex or painful to articulate. The act of creation itself can be a form of release, a way to process and let go of feelings that have been bottled up.

Various forms of artistic expression await your exploration. Painting or drawing can become a window into your soul, where every stroke and color choice reflects your inner world. You don't need to be Van Gogh to find solace in painting. It's about capturing the shades of your emotions, whether it's the bright yellow of hope or the deep blues of melancholy. Writing poetry or short stories offers a narrative outlet where you can weave tales of motherhood, love, and resilience. These stories can be shared or kept private, like little treasures tucked away for when you need them. Engaging in crafts like knitting or scrapbooking allows your hands to work while your mind finds peace. Crafting can be incredibly meditative, providing a rhythmic escape from the chaos of daily life.

Creativity in mental health is more than just a hobby; it's a tool for healing and growth. The focused activity of creating art can have a calming effect, similar to meditation. It draws you into the present moment, away from worries about the past or future. This focus can foster a sense of achievement as you see the fruits of your labor come to life. Even small creative accomplishments can boost confidence, reminding you of your capability to bring beauty into the world.

Integrating creativity into your daily life might seem daunting at first, but small steps can lead to meaningful change. Consider setting up a dedicated creative space at home, even if it's just a corner of a room. Having a place where your supplies are readily available makes it easier to dive into a project whenever inspiration strikes. Scheduling regular art sessions as part of your self-care routine can ensure that creativity becomes a consistent part of your life. These sessions don't have to be lengthy or involved. Even fifteen minutes of sketching or coloring can provide a mental reset, like a mini-vacation for your mind.

Creative Space Checklist

To help you get started, here's a simple checklist: Find a corner in your home where you feel comfortable. Gather your materials— whether it's paints, yarn, or paper. Consider adding elements that inspire you, like music or favorite quotes. Most importantly, allow yourself the freedom to create without judgment.

This chapter has explored the power of creativity as a form of expression and healing. By incorporating art into your life, you open the door to new ways of understanding and processing your emotions. As you continue on your path, remember that each stroke of the brush or loop of yarn is a step toward embracing your unique story. Next, we'll explore how community and support networks can further enrich your journey, offering connection and camaraderie along the way.

CHAPTER 10: HOPE AND EMPOWERMENT

I magine standing at the foot of a mountain, the peak shrouded in mist, a daunting climb ahead. You might feel small, but what if I told you there are paths worn smooth by the footsteps of those who've climbed before you? With each step, they've left behind stories of resilience and triumph. In this chapter, we'll explore these tales of courage—real-life stories of mothers who've navigated the peaks and valleys of postpartum depression. Their journeys remind us that while the climb may be steep, it is possible, and the view from the top offers a new perspective on strength and hope.

10.1 Inspirational Stories: Overcoming PPD

Kentlee's story is one that stands out. After the birth of her child, she found herself trapped in the throes of severe postpartum depression, struggling to eat, sleep, or care for her baby (SOURCE 1). Her days felt like an endless loop of despair, but something shifted when she reached out for help. With the guidance of a psychologist, she learned to recognize her triggers and practiced relaxation techniques. Over time, her well-being improved, and she became an advocate for other mothers facing similar challenges. Kentlee's transformation from despair to advocacy is a testament to the power of seeking help and the resilience that lies within. Her story reminds us that asking for support is not a weakness but a step toward reclaiming your life.

In another narrative, a mother found herself rebuilding relationships after her recovery from postpartum depression. The journey to mending these bonds was not easy. It required patience, understanding, and a willingness to open up about her struggles. Through therapy and support from friends and family, she learned to communicate her needs and emotions better. This openness not only repaired her relationships but also strengthened them. Her story illustrates the healing power of vulnerability and the importance of nurturing connections with those we hold dear. It shows us that recovery doesn't just happen in isolation but flourishes in the company of others.

The transformative experiences of these women often revolve around a pivotal moment—a turning point. For some, it was discovering an effective coping strategy, like mindfulness or journaling, that helped them manage their emotions. For others, it was the realization that professional help was necessary. These moments, though different for each individual, underscore the importance of taking action and seeking support. They serve as reminders that recovery is a process, one that is unique to each person but ultimately achievable with the right tools and support.

Community support plays a crucial role in these recovery journeys. As highlighted in SOURCE 2, being part of a supportive network can significantly impact mental health recovery. Testimonials from peer support groups reveal how sharing experiences with others can provide practical advice, emotional validation, and a sense of belonging. Family and friends also influence the healing process, offering love, encouragement, and a reminder that you are not alone. These connections create a safety net, catching you when you falter and lifting you when you rise.

Reflecting on these stories, find inspiration in your potential for recovery. Believe in your strength and capacity to overcome challenges. Recognize your achievements, no matter how small they may seem, and set personal goals for your recovery. Embrace the idea that you are capable of change and growth. You are not alone in this climb, and with each step, you move closer to the peak. Let these stories be a beacon of hope, guiding you toward a brighter, more empowered future.

10.2 Empowering Self-Awareness: Knowing and Owning Your Journey

Imagine a moment when you finally pause, take a breath, and truly tune into yourself. It's like finding a hidden room in your house filled with insights and revelations about who you are. Self-awareness is that secret space where understanding your triggers and recognizing your strengths can lead to empowered decision-making. When you identify what sets off your anxiety or what lifts your spirits, you gain a roadmap to navigate life's ups and downs with more confidence. Recognizing patterns in your thoughts and behaviors is like being a detective in your own life, solving the mystery of why you react the way you do. This awareness can transform how you approach challenges, turning obstacles into opportunities for growth and change.

To enhance your self-awareness, practical exercises can be your allies. Consider journaling prompts that invite introspection, like reflecting on a recent emotional reaction and what might have triggered it. Or perhaps explore mindfulness exercises that heighten awareness, such as focusing on your breath or the sensations in your body during a quiet moment. These activities create a space for self-reflection, helping you understand your inner world better. As you write or meditate, you might discover new layers to your thoughts and feelings, like peeling an onion to reveal its core. These moments of clarity can be empowering, giving you the tools to manage your mental health with greater ease.

Taking ownership of your path involves setting personal goals and milestones that reflect your aspirations and desires. Think of it as plotting your course on a map, marking the destinations you wish to reach. Creating a personal mission statement can be a powerful exercise, a guiding light that reminds you of your values and purpose. This statement becomes your anchor, something to return to when you feel adrift. It's about actively participating in your recovery, acknowledging that while some aspects might be beyond your control, there's much that you can influence. By setting goals and crafting a mission statement, you reclaim agency over your life, steering it toward what truly matters to you.

The benefits of self-awareness extend far beyond the immediate moment, contributing to long-term well-being. When you build a toolkit of personal coping strategies, you equip yourself to handle whatever life throws your way. Recognizing early signs of stress or relapse becomes second nature, allowing you to address issues before they escalate. This foresight acts like an early warning system, empowering you to take preventive measures and maintain balance. Self-knowledge fosters resilience, helping you bounce back from setbacks with grace and determination. It's a lifelong companion, guiding you through the ever-changing landscape of life and offering insights and wisdom when you need them most.

Self-Reflection Exercise

Set aside a few quiet moments to consider what truly matters to you. What are your core values? How do they shape your decisions and actions? Write these reflections down, allowing them to guide you in creating a personal mission statement. Let this statement serve as your compass, directing you toward a future aligned with your deepest beliefs and aspirations.

10.3 Building a Resilient Mindset: Strength in Adversity

Picture resilience as a rubber band. Stretch it all you want, and it still snaps back into shape. That's the essence of resilience—bouncing back from setbacks, no matter how stretched you feel. In the context of postpartum depression, resilience becomes a vital ally. It's about transforming challenges into stepping stones for growth. Think of it as learning to dance in the rain rather than waiting for the storm to pass. This mindset turns obstacles into opportunities, allowing you to navigate the rocky terrain of early motherhood with a sense of purpose and strength.

Cultivating resilience doesn't happen overnight, but like planting a garden, it flourishes with care and attention. Practicing gratitude and positivity can lay a strong foundation. Start by acknowledging the small joys, like a quiet moment with a cup of tea or a shared giggle with your baby. These moments, though fleeting, can nourish your spirit and remind you of the beauty amidst the chaos. Developing problem-solving skills is another key strategy. When faced with challenges, take a step back and assess the situation. Break it down into manageable parts, and tackle each one with patience and determination. Over time, this approach not only strengthens your problem-solving abilities but also boosts your confidence in handling whatever life throws your way.

Resilience plays a pivotal role in recovering from postpartum depression. It helps maintain motivation during tough times, acting like a lighthouse guiding you through the fog. Think back to past experiences, moments when you overcame adversity. What did you learn? How did you grow? These reflections can provide valuable insights, helping you apply previous lessons to your current situation. As you learn from your past, you enhance your recovery process, armed with the wisdom gained from navigating previous storms. It's about acknowledging your journey, celebrating your resilience, and using it as a springboard to move forward with renewed strength.

Stories of resilience in action can be incredibly inspiring. Consider individuals who have overcome significant obstacles through sheer determination. Their struggles didn't define them; instead, they used adversity as a catalyst for personal growth. One mother who faced a challenging postpartum period found solace in creative expression. She turned her struggles into art, channeling her emotions onto canvas. This creative outlet became a source of healing and empowerment. Another individual, who encountered numerous setbacks, chose to view each one as a lesson. With time, she transformed her adversities into opportunities for growth, ultimately emerging stronger and more self-assured.

Embracing a resilient mindset doesn't mean ignoring difficulties or pretending they don't exist. It means facing them head-on with courage and determination. By practicing gratitude, honing problem-solving skills, and learning from the past, you build the mental and emotional fortitude needed to thrive. Remember, resilience isn't about being unbreakable; it's about being able to bend without snapping. As you navigate the challenges of motherhood, let resilience be your guiding light, a source of strength that empowers you to rise above adversity and embrace the beauty of the journey.

10.4 Preparing for the Future: Strategies for Long-Term Well-being

Picture this: the whirlwind of early motherhood has settled, and you're finally catching your breath. Now, it's time to think about the long-term—beyond the immediate pressures of postpartum life. Establishing routine mental health check-ins is a fantastic way to keep tabs on your emotional well-being. Consider these check-ins like regular oil changes for your mind, ensuring everything runs smoothly. Whether it's a weekly meditation session or a monthly chat with a therapist, these moments of reflection can help you stay grounded. Continuing with therapy or support groups provides a safe space to navigate new challenges as they arise. These sessions aren't just for crisis moments— they're a way to maintain a healthy mental landscape, much like tending a garden so it flourishes over time.

Looking ahead and setting long-term goals becomes a beacon guiding your path. Creating a personal wellness plan for the next five years might sound ambitious, but it's a way to dream big while staying practical. Think about where you want to be, both personally and professionally. Are there skills you've always wanted to learn or career paths you wish to explore? Identifying these aspirations can provide direction and motivation when life feels aimless. Consider your future mental and emotional health and what steps you can take now to support it. This planning isn't about rigid expectations but rather creating a flexible roadmap that adapts as your life evolves.

Embracing lifelong learning and growth keeps the mind engaged and the spirit vibrant. Engaging in continuous learning opportunities, whether through online courses, workshops, or simply picking up a book, can reignite passions and introduce new ideas. Exploring new hobbies or interests is like opening a door to a world of possibilities. Perhaps you've always wanted to try painting or learn a new language. Letting curiosity guide you can lead to unexpected joys and personal fulfillment. This ongoing development isn't just for career advancement—it's about nurturing a rich inner life that feeds your soul.

Life is full of changes and transitions, and adapting to them with resilience is a valuable skill. Whether you're preparing for the possibility of more children or navigating shifts in your career, having strategies in place can ease the process. Embrace the chaos of family changes with humor and flexibility. Each new addition or shift in dynamics offers a chance to strengthen family bonds and grow together. When it comes to career transitions, approach them with an open mind. This could be an opportunity to reassess your goals and align your professional life with your personal values. Being adaptable doesn't mean letting go of your dreams; it's about finding new ways to pursue them despite life's twists and turns.

As you map out the future, remember that these strategies are not about controlling every aspect but about laying a foundation for stability and growth. They give you the tools to navigate whatever comes your way, ensuring that your mental health remains a priority. Each step you take toward long-term well-being is an investment in yourself that pays dividends in peace, fulfillment, and resilience. So, embrace the possibilities with open arms and a hopeful heart, knowing that the future is yours to shape.

10.5 Encouraging Hope: A Positive Path Forward

Imagine starting your day with a simple affirmation: "Today, I choose hope." This small yet powerful phrase can set the tone for your day. Hope is a bit like that first cup of coffee in the morning— it wakes you up to possibilities and energizes you to face whatever comes your way. In the realm of mental health, hope isn't just wishful thinking. It's a vital ingredient for change and growth. Think of it as the light at the end of a long tunnel, guiding you through darkness. Scientific advances continue to shed light on mental health care, offering new treatments and therapies that bring hope to countless individuals. These breakthroughs are a testament to human resilience and the belief that better days are always within reach.

Maintaining a positive outlook during recovery can be transformative. It's not about ignoring the challenges but rather about nurturing the belief that improvement is possible. When you foster a mindset of possibility, you open doors you never knew existed. Visualization can be a particularly powerful tool. Picture yourself in a future where peace and contentment are your constant companions. This mental imagery is like planting seeds in the garden of your mind, allowing the ideas of what could be to grow and flourish. By focusing on what you want to achieve, you slowly build a path toward those goals, step by step.

To cultivate hope, consider incorporating activities that

encourage optimism into your daily routine. Creating a vision board can be a fun and inspiring exercise. Gather images, quotes, and symbols that represent your dreams and aspirations. Arrange them on a board to create a visual map of your future. This board becomes a tangible reminder of what you're working toward. Practicing daily gratitude exercises can also shift your perspective. Each day, take a moment to acknowledge something you're thankful for. These small reflections can transform your outlook, helping you focus on abundance rather than scarcity.

Stories of hope and perseverance abound, each offering a unique glimpse into the power of the human spirit. Take, for instance, the tale of a woman who, against all odds, found her way through the maze of postpartum depression. Her journey was filled with unexpected triumphs, like rediscovering joy through painting or finding solace in the laughter of her child. These stories remind us that even in the face of adversity, hope can light the way. Another account tells of enduring hope through challenges, where setbacks were met with unwavering determination. These narratives serve as beacons of encouragement, showing that while the path may be rocky, it leads to a place of strength and renewal.

Hope is not merely an abstract concept; it's a force that can propel you forward. By embracing hope, you allow yourself to envision a future filled with possibilities. It's about finding the courage to believe in yourself and your ability to overcome obstacles. Let hope be the melody that accompanies you through each day, a constant reminder that brighter tomorrows await. As you continue on this path, hold onto hope as a companion, guiding you toward a life of fulfillment and joy.

10.6 Your Journey Ahead: Embracing Empowerment and Growth

Imagine for a moment standing at the crossroads of your life, with paths stretching out in all directions. Each path represents a choice, an opportunity, a chance to celebrate who you are and what you've achieved. Embracing your path with confidence means recognizing your personal strengths and achievements. It's about looking back at the mountains you've climbed and the storms you've weathered and realizing that those experiences have shaped you into the resilient person you are today. Each success, no matter how small, is a testament to your determination and courage. This celebration of self is not just a reflection of where you've been but a springboard into the future, where setting bold, empowering goals becomes a thrilling adventure. These goals act as beacons, guiding you toward a future filled with possibility and growth.

Empowerment is the catalyst for transformative change. It ignites a spark within that encourages you to take initiative in both your personal and professional life. It's about stepping into the driver's seat and charting your course with intention. You might find empowerment in little things, like deciding to take up a new hobby or pursuing a passion you've put on hold. Or perhaps it's about making a career move that aligns with your values. Whatever form it takes, empowerment is about making choices that reflect your true self. Alongside this personal growth, building a supportive community of like-minded individuals becomes crucial. These connections provide encouragement and accountability, creating a network where ideas are shared and dreams are nurtured. Surround yourself with those who celebrate your victories and support you through challenges, and you'll find that empowerment becomes a shared experience, a collective journey toward a brighter future.

Fostering a lifelong path of growth requires continuous self-improvement and development. Engage in lifelong learning and education to expand your horizons. Seek out mentors or role models who inspire you and offer guidance. These individuals can provide insights, share experiences, and help you navigate the complexities of life. Whether it's through formal education or simply learning from those around you, each new piece of knowledge adds to the tapestry of your understanding. Growth is not a destination but a constant evolution, a journey without end. It's about being open to change, embracing new perspectives, and allowing yourself the grace to make mistakes and learn from them.

Giving back to others is a powerful way to reinforce your own growth and empowerment. Share your experiences and support others on similar paths by volunteering in mental health advocacy or mentoring new mothers facing postpartum challenges. These acts of kindness and support create ripples that extend far beyond your immediate circle, touching lives in ways you may never fully realize. By offering guidance and encouragement to others, you reinforce the lessons you've learned, and in doing so, you continue to grow. The act of giving becomes a cycle of empowerment, where each person you uplift strengthens the community as a whole.

As you step forward, remember that your journey is uniquely yours, filled with endless opportunities for empowerment and growth. Celebrate each step, learn from each stumble, and embrace the path ahead with confidence. Your story is still unfolding, and the best chapters are yet to come.

CONCLUSION

As you close this book, imagine yourself standing at the edge of a new beginning—a moment where the fog starts to lift, and the path ahead becomes clearer. Throughout these chapters, we've journeyed together through the complexities of postpartum depression, exploring its depths and discovering the many ways to navigate this often-challenging landscape.

We began with an understanding of postpartum depression, distinguishing it from the baby blues and recognizing the importance of early identification. From there, we delved into the emotional rollercoaster that many new mothers experience, acknowledging that these feelings are both valid and manageable. We explored the biological and hormonal factors at play and dispelled the myths surrounding postpartum depression, emphasizing that it is not a sign of weakness but a medical condition requiring care and attention.

Each chapter built upon the last, offering practical strategies for self-assessment, seeking help, and involving partners in the journey. We discussed the importance of building a support network, finding your "mama tribe," and utilizing both professional and peer support. The book also highlighted the significance of maintaining your identity amidst motherhood, managing the emotional load, and finding ways to balance personal and parental roles.

Key takeaways from this book include the power of self-awareness and the necessity of a robust support network. Practical coping strategies—like mindfulness, nutrition, and exercise—are tools to aid you on this path. We also underscored the importance of engaging your partner in your journey, as well as embracing diverse perspectives to enrich your understanding of postpartum experiences.

Writing this book has been deeply personal for me. As a mother of two young boys, I know firsthand the challenges that come with the early stages of motherhood. Reflecting on my journey with postpartum depression, I realized that sharing these experiences is a vital part of my healing process. My hope is that this book provides you with both comfort and guidance, helping to ease some of the stress and anxieties you may encounter.

Above all, I want to leave you with a message of hope and empowerment. Recovery is not just a possibility; it's a reality waiting to unfold. You are not alone in this journey. With each step forward, you reclaim a piece of yourself, moving closer to a life filled with balance and joy.

I encourage you to take the first steps toward implementing the strategies we've discussed. Consider joining a support group or starting a journaling practice. Have that open, honest conversation with your partner about your needs. Each small action is a building block on the path to recovery.

I also invite you to engage with a community of supportive mothers. Share your story, learn from others, and continue to grow together. Look for online forums or local meet-ups where you can connect with others who understand what you're going through.

Thank you for trusting me with your time and allowing this book to be a part of your journey. It takes immense courage to face and address postpartum depression, and I commend you for your commitment to personal growth. Your strength and determination are truly inspiring.

As you move forward, envision a future where postpartum depression is openly discussed and supported. Become an advocate for yourself and others. Help reduce stigma and promote mental health awareness. Together, we can create a world where every mother feels understood and supported.

Remember, you are capable of incredible things. You are not defined by your struggles but by the strength you show in overcoming them. Here's to a future filled with hope, healing, and happiness.

SOURCES

1.   Baby blues after pregnancy | March of Dimes https://www.marchofdimes.org/find-support/topics/postpartum/baby-blues-after-pregnancy#:~:text=The%20symptoms%20of%20postpartum%20depression,suddenly%20decreases%2C%20causing%20mood%20swings.

2.   Nurturing Your Creative Business: Insights from Black Creatives. https://theblackrise.com/nurturing-mental-and-emotional-well-being-a-guide-to-self-compassion-and-self-care-for-black-individuals/

3.   The Risks of Online Gambling - ichinose-hotaru.com. https://ichinose-hotaru.com/?p=1023

4.   Digital Ad Strategy | Runn Media. https://runnmedia.com/digital-ad-strategy/

5.   Association between sleep quality and postpartum depression https://pmc.ncbi.nlm.nih.gov/articles/PMC5322694/

6.   (2016). Australia: Producers need to get ready now for nature's worst. MENA Report, (), n/a.

7.   What's Wrong with the 'Rock Bottom' Approach - Wolf Creek Recovery. https://wolfcreekrecovery.com/blog/whats-wrong-rock-bottom-approach/

8.   The Impact of Parental Involvement on Math Skills | Balades Moto 3034. https://balades-moto-30-34.com/5131-the-impact-of-parental-involvement-on-math-skills-11/

9.   Impact of Digital Currencies on Traditional Banking - Khubsoorat Collection: Latest Tech News, Reviews & Innovations. https://khubsooratcollection.com/impact-of-digital-currencies-on-traditional-banking/

10.   6 Selfish Things People Do in Relationships | Things That Make People Go Aww. https://thingsthatmakepeoplegoaww.com/6-selfish-things-people-do-

in-relationships/

11.   The Goal We're Tired of Setting (and Why We Shouldn't Be) - Propel Women. https://www.propelwomen.org/content/the-goal-were-tired-of-setting-and-why-we-shouldnt-be/gjebiq

12.   Benefits of Getting a Behavior Specialist. https://www.dooleycorpcoaching.com/post/benefits-of-getting-a-behavior-specialist

13.   A Guide to Improve Your Marriage and Overall Family Life - Orange Cova. https://www.orangecova.com/tips-to-improve-your-marriage/

14.   Couples Addiction Help Near Scottsdale, Arizona | Local Treatment. https://couplesrehab.com/scottsdale-a-haven-for-couples-seeking-addiction-help/

15.   Postpartum depression - Symptoms and causes https://www.mayoclinic.org/diseases-conditions/postpartum-depression/symptoms-causes/syc-20376617

16.   Stigma Hinders Treatment For Postpartum Depression https://www.npr.org/2011/08/01/138830120/stigma-hinders-treatment-for-postpartum-depression

17.   Edinburgh Postnatal Depression Scale (EPDS) https://med.stanford.edu/content/dam/sm/ppc/documents/DBP/EDPS_text_added.pdf

18.   Barriers to help-seeking for postpartum depression ... https://www.frontiersin.org/journals/global-womens-health/articles/10.3389/fgwh.2024.1335437/full

19.   Weekly Online Support Group | Join a Free Group Today https://www.postpartum.net/get-help/psi-online-support-meetings/

20.   Peer Support Interventions for Perinatal Depression https://womensmentalhealth.org/posts/essential-reads-peer-support-interventions-for-perinatal-depression/

21.   The Benefits of Attending Support Groups for New Moms https://www.readynestcounseling.com/post/the-benefits-of-attending-support-groups-for-new-moms

22.   How to support your partner through postpartum ... https://www.mavenclinic.com/post/

how-to-support-your-partner-through-postpartum-depression-and-anxiety

23.   Peanut - Find Friends and Support https://www.peanut-app.io/

24.   Effects of family relationship and social support on the mental ... https://bmcpregnancychildbirth.biomedcentral.com/articles/10.1186/s12884-022-04392-w

25.   Mindfulness Techniques for New Mothers: Cultivating Calm   ...   https://www.theholisticcounseling.center/blog/motherhood/mindfulness-techniques-for-new-mothers

26.   Nutritional factors and cross-national postpartum depression ... https://www.frontiersin.org/journals/psychiatry/articles/10.3389/fpsyt.2023.1193490/full#:~:text=Several%20studies%20have%20found%20that,are%20both%20associated%20with%20decreased

27.   Postpartum Workout Plan: 8 At-Home Exercises https://www.healthline.com/health/postpartum-workout-plan

28.   Insomnia and Postpartum Depression: Sleep Tips for New Moms   https://www.michiganmedicine.org/health-lab/insomnia-and-postpartum-depression-when-new-moms-sleep-loss-turns-perilous#:~:text=Fortunately%2C%20we%20have%20good%20treatments,changing%20behaviors%20to%20improve%20sleep.

29.   Identity   Shift   In   Motherhood   https://councilforrelationships.org/identity-shift-in-motherhood-navigating-new-challenges-rediscovering-yourself/

30.   Finding Balance Between Personal Identity and Parenting https://easypeasie.com/blogs/peapod-blog/celebrating-motherhood-finding-balance-between-personal-identity-and-parenting#:~:text=By%20making%20self%2Dcare%20a,of%20health%20and%20well%2Dbeing.

31.   Carrying the Mental Load: How to Redistribute the Burden ... https://momwell.com/blog/carrying-the-mental-load-how-to-redistribute-the-burden-and-give-moms-more-freedom

32.   Mom Guilt: Causes & 13 Tips for Overcoming https://www.choosingtherapy.com/mom-guilt/

33.   Associations Between Spousal Relationship, Husband ... https://www.ncbi.nlm.nih.gov/pmc/articles/PMC8966113/

34.   Effective   Communication   Strategies for   Couples   https://epiccounselingsolutions.com/effective-communication-strategies-for-couples-a-therapists-guide/

35.   How   Equally   Shared   Parenting   Benefits   Child and   Parent   https://www.dcomply.com/how-equally-shared-parenting-benefits-child-and-parent/

36.   Communication and Intimacy Tools for New Parents https://www.psychologytoday.com/us/blog/preparing-for-parenthood/202303/communication-and-intimacy-tools-for-new-parents#:~:text=Couples%20who%20understand%20each%20other's,will%20improve%20the%20emotional%20connection.

37.   The Impact of Cultural Factors Upon Postpartum Depression   https://www.tandfonline.com/doi/full/10.1080/07399330802089149

38.   Overcoming The Stigma of Maternal Mental Health: Why It ... https://ppdil.org/2024/01/overcoming-the-stigma-of-maternal-mental-health/

39.   Culturally Responsive Care in Mental Health https://www.lyrahealth.com/resources/culturally-responsive-care/

40.   "just   like   therapy!":   Investigating   the   Potential   of Storytelling ... https://arxiv.org/pdf/2212.03452

41.   Researchers   Confirm   Postpartum   Depression Heritability,   ...   https://news.unchealthcare.org/2023/10/researchers-confirm-postpartum-depression-heritability-home-in-on-treatment-mechanism/

42.   Interpersonal Psychotherapy for Postpartum Depression - PMC   https://pmc.ncbi.nlm.nih.gov/articles/PMC4141636/#:~:text=At%20present%2C%20interpersonal%20psychotherapy%20is,especially%20for%20depressed%20breastfeeding%20women.

43.   10 Best Apps To Deal With Postpartum Depression https://www.calmsage.com/best-apps-to-deal-with-postpartum-depression/

44.   How to Find a Postpartum Depression Therapist You Can ... https://www.whattoexpect.com/first-year/postpartum-health-and-care/postpartum-depression-therapist

45.   Evaluation of expressive writing for postpartum health https://pmc.ncbi.nlm.nih.gov/articles/PMC6209049/#:~:text=Another%20study%20using%20a%20variation,(Di%20Blasio%20et%20al.%2C

46.   Creative Outlets for Recovery from Depression https://www.webmd.com/depression/depression-creative-outlets

47.   105 Self Reflect Questions For New Moms to Ask Themselves https://char-dion.com/self-reflect-questions/

48.   Screening Tools for Postpartum Depression and Anxiety https://whatcomperinatal.org/perinatal-screening-tools/

49.   Postpartum Depression: Kentlee's Story https://www.hopkinsmedicine.org/health/wellness-and-prevention/postpartum-mood-disorders-what-new-moms-need-to-know/patient-story-kentlee

50.   The Role of Community Support in Mental Health Recovery https://www.fundamentalchange.life/the-role-of-community-support-in-mental-health-recovery

51.   Build Self-Awareness: Ten Self-Reflection Exercises and ... https://www.lumiacoaching.com/blog/self-awareness-tools

52.   Managing Your Loved One's Health Better. https://angelshomecareprovider.com/managing-your-loved-ones-health-better

53.   Postpartum care tips for new mothers | TheHealthSite.com. https://www.thehealthsite.com/pregnancy/pregnancy-guide-pregnancy/postpartum-care-things-you-can-do-to-make-your-motherhood-journey-simpler-943137/

54.   Resilience and mental health among perinatal women - NCBI https://www.ncbi.nlm.nih.gov/pmc/articles/PMC11298415/#:~:text=As%20identified%20in%20different%20literature,environment%20(20%E2%80%9322).

55.   Unlocking the Power of Effective Communication in English Conversations. https://www.edyoufest.org/post/unlocking-the-power-of-effective-communication-in-english-

conversations

56.   The Benefits of Professional Grief Counseling - Houston Funeral Guide. https://houstonfuneralguide.com/the-benefits-of-professional-grief-counseling/

57.   The Benefits of Professional Grief Counseling - Houston Funeral Guide. https://houstonfuneralguide.com/the-benefits-of-professional-grief-counseling/

58.   3 Reasons To Seek Out A Primary Care Physician - About Jessica's Cosmetic Surgeries. http://jessicagoodyear.com/2016/12/22/3-reasons-to-seek-out-a-primary-care-physician/

59.   With every trial and challenge we face, we need courage and a positive outlook to overcome them - Prayer & Encouragement - Crossmap Communities - Christian Forums. https://communities.crossmap.com/t/with-every-trial-and-challenge-we-face-we-need-courage-and-a-positive-outlook-to-overcome-them/4795

60.   How To Commit To Putting Your Best Work Out Into The World - Merce Cardus. https://mercecardus.com/how-to-commit-to-putting-your-best-work-out-into-the-world/

61.   Unlocking the Power of Effective Communication in English Conversations. https://www.edyoufest.org/post/unlocking-the-power-of-effective-communication-in-english-conversations

62.   Beautifully put! - Janice Tovey - Medium. https://1birthdayfun.medium.com/beautifully-put-e1c1a57fe861

63.   Tricia Chandler, Rapid Transformational Therapy and Trauma Coaching. https://www.triciachandler.com/

64.   The Process of Mindful Arts Therapy - Mindful Arts Therapy. https://mindfulartstherapy.com.au/the-process-of-mindful-arts-therapy/

65.   Cultivating Mindfulness Through Journaling: A Gateway to Inner Peace - Lid: AI-Powered Voice Journaling. https://www.getlid.co/cultivating-mindfulness-through-journaling-a-gateway-to-inner-peace/

66.   Navigating Parenthood How a Postpartum Depression Therapist Can Make a Difference - entrepreneursprohub. https://entrepreneursprohub.com/navigating-parenthood-how-a-postpartum-depression-therapist-can-make-a-difference/

Made in the USA
Monee, IL
28 May 2025

aff12a51-7f34-421d-9f95-88b864f9a0b7R01